"A physician shares his trials with chronic pain in this debut medical memoir…For those dealing with chronic pain while reading Moody's astute, candid, and thoughtful guide—packed with helpful charts and uncredited black-and-white illustrations—there is nothing superfluous in these pages. Using a conversational tone and keeping his text readable and easily digestible by a general audience, the author articulates and compassionately relates to the seemingly endless struggle to overcome physical pain and carry on with daily life. While some chapters offer valuable information, medical guidance, and hopeful, reassuring advice, others are more practical and directly address the frank reality and discouraging aspects of living with chronic pain. Some readers may ponder what Moody really means when he admits to remaining in pain but accepting it and no longer suffering from it. But his 'pain willingness' process explains this epiphany in the book's conclusion…A useful and illuminating guide that encourages a greater awareness of a crippling syndrome affecting legions of patients."
—*Kirkus Reviews*

I0481128

Moody, H. (a pseudonym)
Truce! A Physician Makes Peace with Chronic Pain

ISBN: 1—9816—1132—0

First Edition

For my parents,
who have felt every twinge.

Table of Contents

I. The Pain Begins

Doctor Heal Thyself   8
Your Body's Language   12
The Doctor-Patient Relationship   16
Diagnosis, Diagnosis, Diagnosis   20
Collecting the Evidence   26
The Chronic Pain Syndrome   34
The Pain-Prone Patient   44
Flex the Complex, Break the Brittle   50

II. Treating the Pain

First, Do No Harm   58
Evidence Based Medicine   68
Five Common Diagnosis   78
Down the Rabbit Hole   86
The Opioid Escalator   94
Alchemy   104
Team Treatment   114
Have Scalpel, Will Travel   122
What If This Is As Good As It Gets?   130
Alternative Treatments   134

III. Now What?

When is Enough, Enough?   144
You Find Out Who Your Friends Are   150
The Disability Treadmill   156
Dark Night of the Soul   162
Escaping the Rabbit Hole   166
Pain Willingness   170
End-notes   174

I. The Pain Begins

"On a day when I start to sink into that 'Why me?' mood, I turn it into 'Why not me?' I, too, have health insurance. I, too, did not suffer financially when I had to stop working.... I, too, have the best of caregivers. So why not me?"

—Toni Bernhard, *How to be Sick*

Doctor Heal Thyself

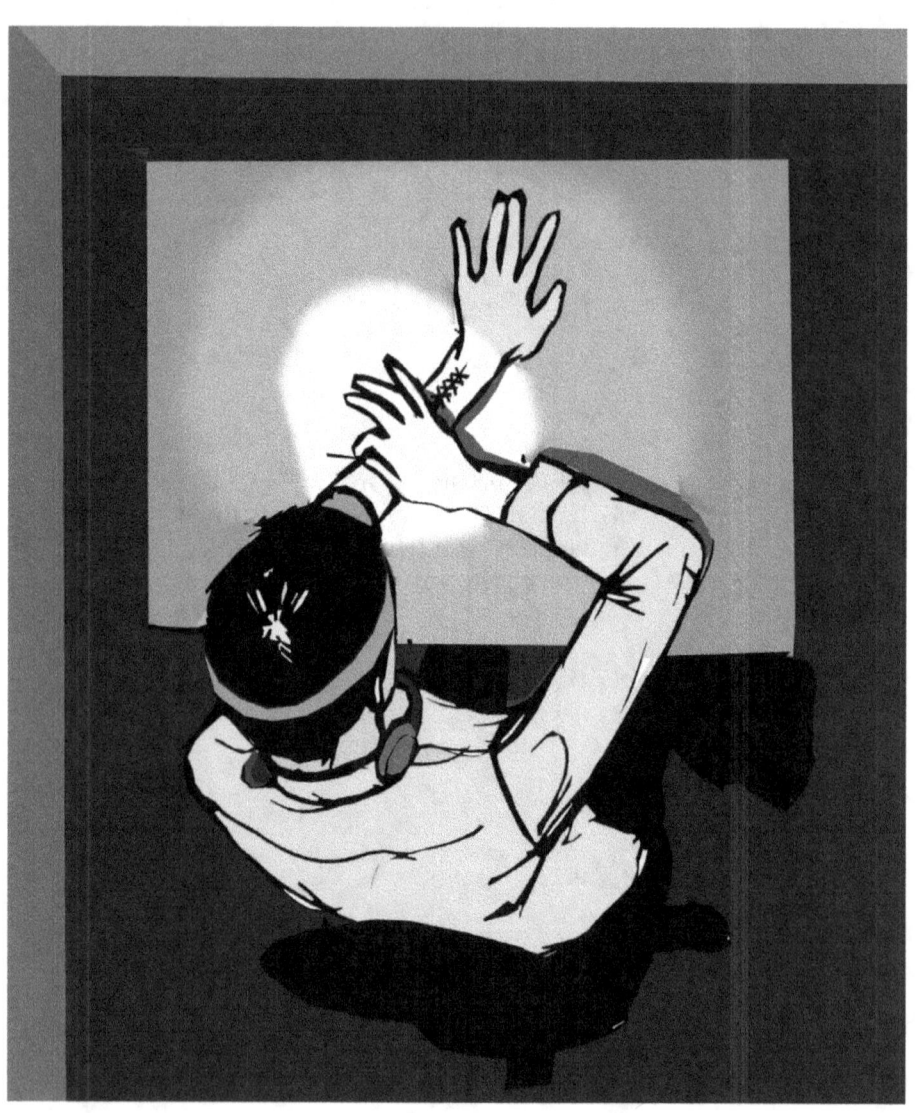

"The doctor is effective only when he himself is affected. Only the wounded physician heals."

—Carl Jung

Write about what you know.

Not about what you've studied in the library for months and think you know, or even what you know better than many others, but what you truly know. Unfortunately (for writers) 99% of things are already known, and written about; but 1% of people live extraordinary lives, and a subgroup of them rise above the others. My extraordinariness is not talent related, but circumstantial—wrong person, wrong place, wrong time.

I know pain. Not the pain of heartache or a skinned knee, but the rare type that never goes away. Pain that uproots life, forces disability and ends relationships. This gets me into the 1%, but not what floats me to the top— that singularity is that I am also a pain doctor. I am a pain doctor with chronic pain.

You've heard the anecdote before, the doctor suffering from the disease he treats. A cardiologist having a heart attack, or a pulmonologist with lung cancer. Well, I am an anesthesiologist; so I oblige, follow tradition and suffer my specialty—pain, and its relief.

Anesthesiologists strategize; we don't just flip a switch. We anticipate where the scalpel will cut and inject numbing medicine, deadening those nerves to the blade. We guide long needles into pregnant backs—cursed on the way in, blessed on the way out—and we shepherd the mind through surgery by titrating the depth of unconsciousness (too deep an ending, too light an awakening, which is worse?). Anesthesia is checking, and double checking, all...day...long. We prepare for catastrophe, setting up machines and medications needed three chess moves into the future, then put it all away, unused and unappreciated (today).

But no foresight prepared me for the calamity heading my way, no numbing medicine deadened my nerves when the pain began, and no ether drifted me to sleep. I was awake when the scalpel cut—I'm awake!—but nobody cared; students became residents, residents became doctors and hospital life moved on. But the pain seemed to care, it stayed.

I became the doctor-patient, a hybrid with access and knowledge. I ordered x-rays and then jumped into the machine, checked off blood tests and rolled up my own sleeve. No one noticed the physician and patient bore the same name; no one notices anything when you wear a white lab coat.

Despite the inside track I was misdiagnosed and mistreated. My colleagues made themselves scarce, and the pain grew worse, continually worse. A decade later, as a physician and chronic pain patient, I have all the literature on pain weighing down my bookshelf. There are journal articles for doctors, memoirs for patients, books on rare and general illnesses and even a series written by patients for doctors. But where are the books by rheumatologists with arthritis, or neurosurgeons with brain cancer?

Well, I've poked a lot of patients with needles, and been poked a lot myself, feeling the sharp objects of my trade from both sides. I've prescribed, and popped, every available pain medication. I've had four spine operations, and performed anesthesia for hundreds of others. Yes, I know the spectrum of treatments for chronic pain. So I write this missing manual to fill a void— a book on pain, by a pain doctor, in pain.

I am not a writer by trade, but learnt this craft to write this magnum opus (there will be no volume two). I'm a carpenter that will build one table. This isn't a five-steps-to-being-pain-free type self-help book, but observations from someone who hurts all the time, along with explanations of medications, procedures and diagnosis. Anecdotes mixed with medical evidence, in plain language. My ideal readers haven't aged into pain, but have had it prematurely thrust upon them, and are somewhere amidst the procedures, medications and surgeries by the time this book lands in their lap. I've lived the other side, but am a turn-coat and look at life through a patient's eyes now.

There are three sections: the flurry after the pain begins; the flurry as the pain is treated; and the calm after the hustle and bustle is done. Five chapters are noticeably different because they explore the philosophical side of pain, and outline my roadmap to a happy ending: I remain in pain, but no longer suffer from pain. I don't promise my steps can be re-trodden, but by way of your own path you can reach the same destination—acceptance of pain.

Acceptance allows us to be present with pain, and move on with life. The pain lives on, but in the background as white noise, and the suffering goes. As folding laundry, grocery shopping and taking the dog for a walk are second nature to living, so too managing pain becomes routine and commonplace. Instead of the vortex around which everything swirls, it's another to-do on a crumpled list of errands in our pocket.

Anyone with pain will benefit from reading this book, but the enormity of the topic called for some winnowing. T.S. Eliot once wrote, "If I had more time, I would have written a shorter letter"—it is with that sentiment that I offer this slim book. I took the time—I read the doorstoppers and sieved the studies—and conclude: little is known, little is understood, little is proven. Chronic pain is an orphan diagnosis, in all ways except prevalence. The choosing and excluding that was left was done by I the patient, not I the physician. How much personal narrative versus clinical approach? How much horribleness versus encouragement? The chapters reach to both ends of the spectrum, the cheery and discouraging, and are midway between the two extremes of books on pain: the overly technical and the overly spiritual.

More women suffer chronic pain than men, so I assign my generic patient the pronouns she and her. And more working physicians are still men, so I assign my generic doctor the pronouns he and him, thus splitting the pronouns and avoiding confusion. But mostly it'll be you and I, as we are on this journey together.

Patients go through five stages as they grieve a terminal illness; I define four stages chronic pain patients go through on their way to acceptance. But there are stark differences because we are not terminal, but have a disease that's interminable, and this missing endpoint is why so few of us make it to the final stage of acceptance. We stutter at each step, hoping to regress to our old lives, but as we wait we fail to progress, because we see this as the wrong direction. It took me a decade to figure this out; to turn the rearview mirror to the roof and drive onward into the night.

Maybe tomorrow we'll wake up without pain.

Your Body's Language

"Pain is a more terrible lord of mankind than even death itself."

—Dr. A. Schweitzer, 1931

The day my pain began I was playing tennis. For forehands and backhands you're meant to turn your feet sideways to hit the ball, but I discovered keeping my feet facing the net, and twisting my torso, I could hit the ball and return to my ready position faster. I was in a competitive game, and thanks to adrenaline I felt no pain as I twisted harder with each stroke of the racquet. The next morning I awoke with burning in my left buttock: it was red, hot and swollen.

Inflammation

Years before residency training, the first lecture of medical school taught the body's response to injury, its language: inflammation. It was described first in Latin as rubor, tumor, calor and dolor which translates to redness, swelling, heat and pain. These four signs of inflammation are the body's means of communicating harm, and of healing itself. Signs are visible or measureable manifestations of a disease (fever); symptoms are invisible and not measureable (feeling nausea). Inflammation lets you know you've a pulled a muscle, torn a ligament or bruised a knee; scrape your arm and you'll see redness, this is inflammation.

As injury occurs, the arteries and veins send out signals for help; these blood vessels become leaky, and blood shifts from the space inside the vessel to the space outside the vessel, where the injury occurred. This relocation of blood causes the swelling, redness and heat, and as pain receptors in the skin are compressed the final component, pain. Pain alerts the mind to the injury, while the blood heals the damage. White blood cells treat infection; platelets stop bleeding; red blood cells haul oxygen (the body's food) to organs and carbon dioxide (the body's trash) to the lungs. The body heals its daily injuries with us none the wiser.

At the cellular level of all disease is inflammation, indicated by the suffix –itis, which means "inflamed." Arthritis, appendicitis, meningitis, hepatitis, dermatitis, sinusitis, colitis, gastritis, esophagitis, tonsillitis, pancreatitis etc. Inflammation is curative: the pain causes us to safeguard the injury, while the blood does its job of repair. But excessive swelling causes problems in areas where there is no room to expand (we drill holes into the skull to relieve brain swelling).

Anti-Inflammatories

My ill-advised tennis moves caused pain and swelling, warning me in a language I was fluent to take it easy. But I was young and thought myself bulletproof, and reached for the most commonly used medication in the world, over-the-counter non-steroidal anti-inflammatory drugs (NSAIDs henceforth). It was some brand of Advil (ibuprofen), Aleve (naproxen) or aspirin (I capitalize brand or trade names, and use lowercase for generic drug names). NSAIDs reduce swelling and ease pain, but if the underlying diagnosis is untreated they only mask symptoms, silencing alarms unheeded. My current regimen is to take 800mg of ibuprofen at night before going to sleep, and none throughout the day. This allows my body to benefit from the curative anti-inflammatory effects, but not mask my body's pain response throughout the day.

Some inflammation is so severe NSAIDs fail, and prescription-strength steroidal anti-inflammatory drugs are needed (prednisone). Asthmatics inhale steroids into their lungs, patients with dermatitis use steroid creams and arthritis patients are given steroid injections into their joints. Our "steroids" aren't the muscle enlarging compounds (those are anabolic steroids), but these powerful drugs to decrease inflammation. Moving from NSAIDs (non-steroids) to steroids is a sizable step because of the escalating side-effects.

You and I, we are chronic pain patients, and know medications and stoicism only help so much when we hurt. It's better to be attuned to our body's language and avoid flare-ups in the first place. Pain is this language, wrenching our concentration away to address the matter at hand, the source of the pain. Learn this language now; I did so the hard way. With these symptoms—pain, redness, heat and swelling—I should have taken the day off to rest. But I took Ibuprofen, blocked the pain, and played another six hours of tennis. I would never be the same.

Your body's language—inflammation—has but four words to communicate harm: redness, swelling, heat and pain.

The Doctor-Patient Relationship

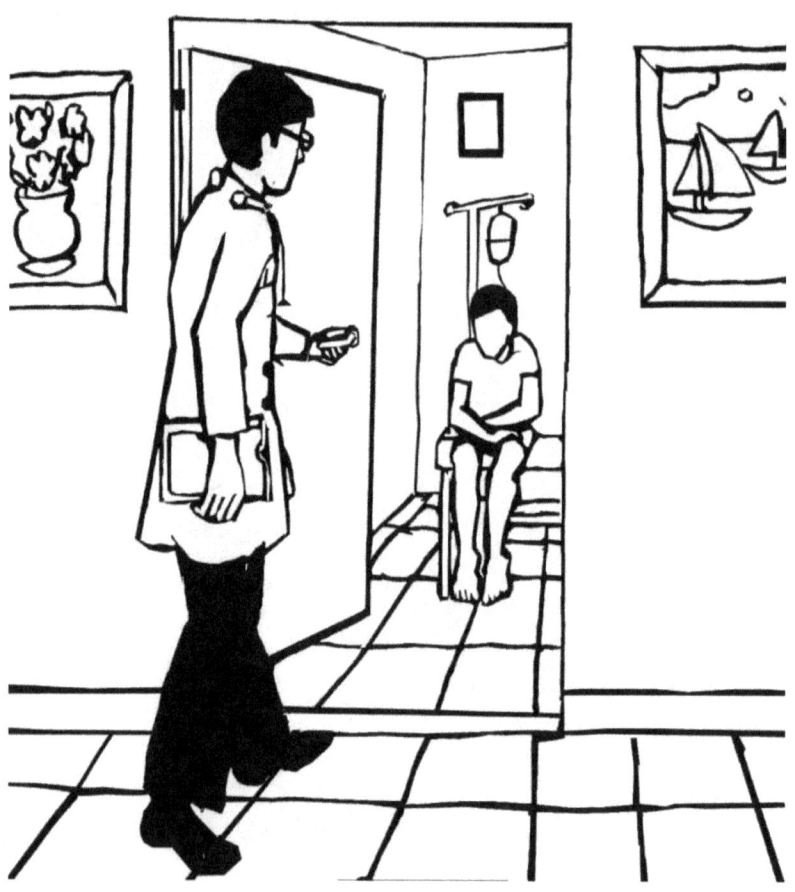

"The patient, who is seeking medical solutions, has placed total responsibility on the physician. The physician has willingly assumed this responsibility but has not kept the implicit agreement to make the patient well again….[T]he physician, who has applied his or her expertise and technical skill in a genuine attempt to treat the problem, may also feel betrayed by the patient. … [who] does not keep his or her end of the implicit agreement by reporting improvements in symptoms."

—*Coping with Chronic Pain*

Primary care doctors are the gateway to treatment. One hundred million Americans a year suffer from pain[1], which is a lot of patients to squeeze through a gateway. Patients expect their primary care doctor to diagnose and treat their pain, and physicians expect to diagnose and treat each patient under their care. This duo, doctor and patient, begin a search for the cause of the pain, with both expecting a diagnosis and treatment to be found. But when the diagnosis is elusive, and acute pain turns chronic, stress is placed on the doctor-patient relationship. The patient then begins a well-delineated journey: disillusionment with her physician, conflicting information from her specialists, conflict over medications and a search for alternative treatments.[2, 3]

The doctor-patient relationship is special. As the door closes, the words become sacrosanct, legally protected from even family member's inquiries. The physical relationship is intimate: no other professional examines you unclothed. You come together with one goal, your health, but the bond extends further: family life, financial problems, relationships and work-life all pass through that clinic room as they take turns affecting your health. Physicians only have three tools to treat patients: the prescription pad, the scalpel and the relationship.[4] The pad and scalpel are overemphasized in our society, and too little emphasis is placed on the healing power of the doctor-patient relationship.

As the relationship deepens you learn your doctor is human, like you. Vulnerable to illness, greed, carelessness and lack of empathy, he'll be hungry the appointment before lunch, and grumpy for the last patient of the day. Doctors get stressed, will cut you off when rushed, and they will disappoint. Every physician starts out noble in medical school, but somewhere during residency, as the hours increase that nobility wanes. Their path delays gratification, with peers earning money, starting businesses, getting married and having children while the resident-doctor slaves away in training, two-hundred thousand dollars in debt. Amidst the student-intern-residency progression, the practice of new procedures, surgeries, lack of sleep and perpetual exams, the treatment of patients becomes automatized. The personal touch is lost to a conveyor-belt progression from room to room.

If your doctor is letting you down, move on. You can't change him into who you want him to be. If a doctor doesn't listen or address your concerns, move on. If it's a struggle to get prescriptions refilled, or disability forms filled in on time, move on. If he doubts your pain because your x-rays are normal, for God's sake, move on.

Finding a Doctor

I have known many doctors, as an anesthesiologist and then a patient: last count I had 32 treating physicians, spanning six specialties and four states. None had answers. Actually, they all had answers, just wrong answers. I got angry with some, exasperated with others and taunted a few. But only when a doctor gets sick and suffers will he understand the trust he holds in his hands. You have no choice but to go to him for help, but you do have a right to demand respect.

My internist helped the most. He said he didn't know the cause of my pain, and his truthfulness set me at ease. We brainstormed together, bouncing ideas off each other. Determined to help, he organized my disabled parking placard, filled my prescriptions and completed disability forms on time. These mundane tasks removed stressors from my life, and lessened my discomfort. He was a team leader, arranging the specialists to act in concert.

When you look for a doctor, separate personality from medical expertise. Amiability, accessibility and organization are qualities to seek in a primary care physician; experience, skill and reputation are qualities to look for in a specialist. Who cares if your surgeon thinks he walks on water, as long as he is a skilled surgeon? To find these experts, figure out who other doctors go to as patients; as only doctors can judge other doctors, and then only if they are of the same specialty. Ask orthopedists who'd operate on them; one name will keep popping up, and this is the surgeon you choose (irrespective of their ill-nature).

Failing to help a patient is hard for a physician. Medicine is founded on science, and doctors thrive when they translate that learning into a cure. Admitting a lack of knowledge stresses the physician, and strains the physician-patient relationship. Confronting your doctor regarding his inability to cure you will cause a defensive reaction, because in those shoes you'd protect yourself from criticism too. He will then take the safer route of passing the buck and referring you along.

Cultivate an alliance with your doctor, strengthening the bond despite a lack of medical progress. Understanding the psychology of the relationship early on allows you to draw your physician closer. Empathize and encourage him, "I know this is hard for you, too," "I understand if this doesn't work," and "I appreciate you trying." He needs to feel blameless for your lack of progress, or regression, to have confidence to attempt treatments with lower chances of success. An experimental surgery fixed me, but only after I brought the surgeon close; over a year's time I assured and reassured him until he was comfortable to cut. I held him blameless before he even operated, and consequently became the test case for his new technique. You may need to pioneer a new treatment, so begin transforming your doctor-patient relationship into a doctor-patient partnership.

Find the quarterback of your team.

Diagnosis, Diagnosis, Diagnosis

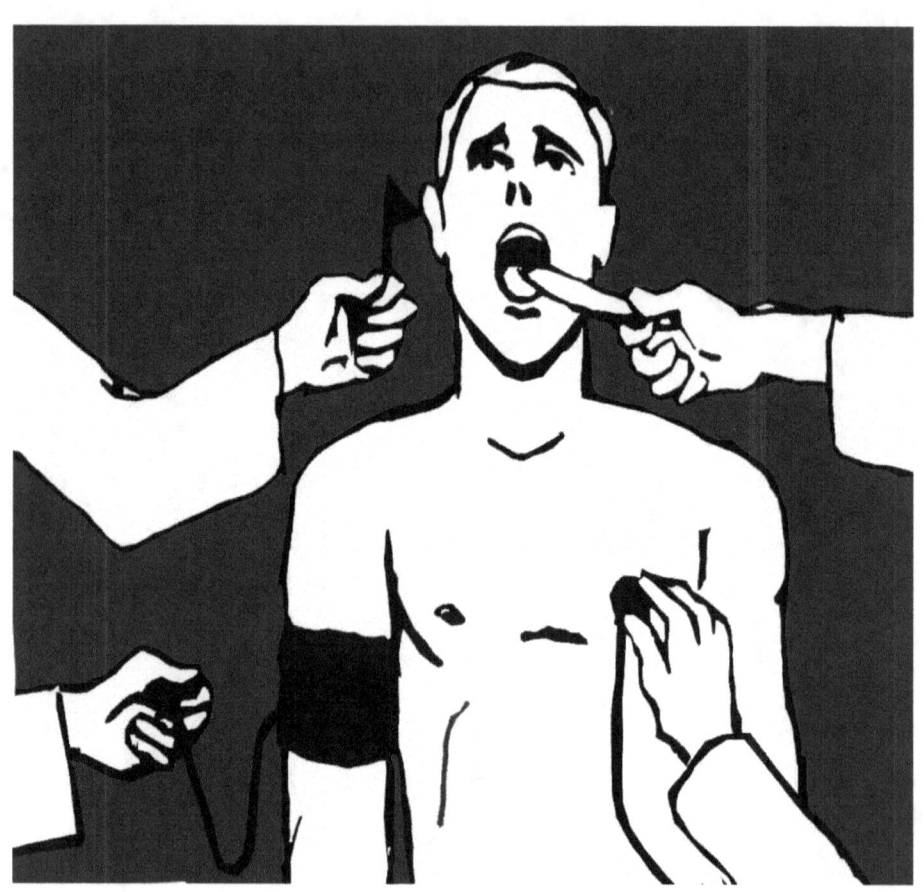

"When pain persists and feels like it is ruining your life, it is difficult to see how it can be serving any purpose. But even when pain is chronic and nasty, it hurts because the brain has somehow concluded, for some reason or another, often completely subconsciously, that you are threatened and in danger—the trick is finding out why the brain has come to this conclusion."

—David Butler, *Explain Pain*

Real estate's motto, "Location, location, location," conveys the same importance as the slogan for chronic pain, "Diagnosis, diagnosis, diagnosis."

Chronic pain is an edgeless jigsaw puzzle, because research has only been funded the last 20 years. But one corner-piece of the puzzle is in hand: once diagnosed you're labeled, linked to a billing code forever. If the label—diagnosis and numeric code—is wrong, all treatments will fail. So allow doubt, question the diagnosis and be suspicious of he who says, "This is surely what's causing your pain."

To see a doctor, have a procedure or fill a prescription a diagnosis has to be listed for billing purposes. A vague diagnosis—"low back pain"—is better than a specific diagnosis—"discogenic back pain"—because the former will keep physicians mindful that the pain's cause is unknown. One secret is to add NOS after your symptom, which means Not Otherwise Specified: Back Pain NOS, Arm Pain NOS and even Chronic Pain NOS are actual billing codes which describe the problem, communicate the cause as unknown and allow insurance billing. It's a wastebasket diagnosis, something to throw patients into who have a symptom without a cause, but remain here as long as possible to keep doctors engaged and thinking.

Pain treatment has no algorithm for "the next step." There are few statistics for improvement or cure, and patients are given an educated guess to the source of their pain (the pain generator). Cancer is the other extreme, with standardized treatment progression—surgery, radiation, chemotherapy—and precise cure rates available. Cancer's progress is tracked by an oncologist, who briefs a radiation oncologist and surgeon on the size and spread of the cancer. When cancer patients go to appointments their next step has already been decided before they arrive. They have the luxury of burying their heads in the sand as they are led along a pathway of treatments.

In sharp contrast, we hop from specialist to specialist, who aren't under a unified umbrella or in contact with one another (and at-times disdain one another). We must act as record keepers between these compartmentalized specialists; we can't bury our heads in the sand, but must become versed in medicalese to understand what's going on. We are the storytellers who must brief the next doctor. There will be no phone conference before our appointments, because who wants to discuss a negative x-ray, failed procedure or ineffective medication?

Americans can't conceive of a disease as untreatable, or unnamed; but if you're reading this book you know the nameless or incurable. Keep track of everything tried—medications, doses, procedures, surgeries and presumed diagnosis—to produce a historical record and avoid backtracking. I carry a one page typed list of procedures, with the dates performed and presumed diagnosis.

A Potpourri of Diagnosis

The burning in my hip didn't go away; I was diagnosed with bursitis, an inflammation of a sac of fluid near the hipbone. I was treated with NSAIDs, steroid injections and finally systemic steroids (prednisone). Then the pain began in my other hip, but the doctors continued to say I had bursitis (of both hips!). I questioned this, refusing to be pigeonholed with an incorrect diagnosis. The swelling and pain marched on to my groin and thighs, and my rheumatologist yielded. I didn't have bursitis.

Doctors went on to misdiagnose me, with great certainty, another seven times: fasciitis, panniculitis, facet-syndrome, discogenic back pain, femoral cutaneous nerve entrapment, posterior-rami syndrome and failed back syndrome. I wasn't correctly diagnosed for seven more years. And not by a doctor.

Categorizing Pain

Pain come in three varieties:

1) Pain with a preceding cause: a car crash, accident or fall.
2) Pain with a confirming test (x-ray, CT, MRI) or visible signs.
3) Pain without a known cause, abnormal test result or external sign.

Patients in categories 1 and 2 will encounter sympathetic practitioners (believers in their pain), who will try harder to treat the visible cause of their pain. Those in category three will fight the triple battle of 1) finding the pain generator, 2) keeping doctors convinced of the authenticity of their pain and 3) obtaining pain relief. But all three categories are a Faustian bargain—a yin and yang—with good accompanying bad. Categories one and two receive the best treatment for their respective causes; they gain pain relief, not a pain cure, and remain chronic pain patients. Those in category three can hope that if diagnosed correctly, treatment will be swift and absolute.

I began in category three, misdiagnosed and mistreated for six years, until a leg length discrepancy was found from a torn ligament. Once correctly diagnosed I transitioned from category 3 to 2: treatment led to swift and wonderful relief, but not a cure. I remain in category 2, with secondary pain diagnosis rooted in my life. Would a correct diagnosis two, four or six years earlier have resulted in a less severe resting point?

Andrew Solomon, when writing[5] about depression, condenses it down to a single word: imminent. For chronic pain our word is: unpredictable. We never know when the pain will flare, knocking us to our beds and putting life on hold. The 1 to 10 pain scale is for hospital, clinical, and medical use; I categorize my pain as a one, two or three; and I associate physical, emotional and intellectual abilities with each level. I don't listen to weather forecasts, but I do look out the window in the morning for sun, rain or snow before getting dressed. Predicting pain is even more uncertain than weather; but dressing correctly for today's weather, or pain, is doable. Associating pain severity with irritability and tolerance levels will let you know which social invitations to accept, what errands to run and how far to travel from home. The only thing worse than getting caught in the rain without an umbrella, is getting caught at a dinner party during a pain flare.

Level 1 pain—on this 1 to 3 scale—is still rotten, but doesn't prevent me from functioning in society. I go out to dinner, grocery shopping and do house-work. It's there every day, but I still do things. This is the lowest my pain gets, and I make decisions on a month-to-month basis. When I'm the least irritable I do the most irritating things: dealing with health insurance companies, visiting the curmudgeon family member, reprogramming my TiVo or strategizing with my pain team. This is also when I do the most social and physically taxing activities.

Level 2 pain is when my daily routine falters. I am housebound, bed-bound, state or city-bound. I set my television up in my bedroom, order my groceries online and hire an assistant. I make plans day-to-day and wouldn't agree to a party one week out. I become impatient easier, so I avoid aggravating things. I get the oil changed in my car, return library books, buy stamps or go to the ATM. I note the direction of movement, ensuring I'm descending to 1, not rising to 3.

Level 3 pain is the flare-up. I get breathless and frantic and suicidal thoughts race through my mind: "Oh my God! It's got to stop!" I'm drowning in water, my arms flailing to find purchase. I hit this level intermittently, bumping up to it before falling back to level 2. It's my ceiling, the worst my pain gets, but not somewhere I live.

Your pain is horrid, I know, so is mine; it's hard to contemplate worse. Work in a pain clinic and you'll see worse, patients living at level 3 every day. Their most common diagnosis is Complex Regional Pain Syndrome (CRPS henceforth): they hurt from a soft touch, a light breeze or a sheet brushing across their skin. What's remarkable isn't their pain, but the slightness of their injuries. One patient bumped her elbow against a door frame, and then like an anaconda enveloping its prey the pain coiled up and down her arm, hand to shoulder. She couldn't cut her fingernails or wear clothing on the affected arm, the pain of the cloth was too great. The hair fell out and the skin turned dark purple as the venom progressed. She wore a tent-like structure, fashioned by her father, suspending the arm in a sensation-free space (an outer skin for the serpent). Yes, pain can get worse.

Quantify your pain as a 1, 2 or 3 and record it daily. Correlate activities to pain levels each day: is there a pattern? When my pain is at a 1, I am more active, but my diary revealed level 3 days frequently followed level 1 days. Bring this pain diary to your pain doc to help adjust your pills and brainstorm together for triggers. This will give credence to your pain, as you try to correlate pain medications to a pain level, and not to get high (no one selling opioids on the street would fake a pain diary). Pain is invisible with no external sign of what's wrong; the depressed have the same annoyance, even self-mutilating themselves to bring the physical state in-line with the mental.[6]

The 1-10 pain scale is patient specific, and better evaluates changes due to a new medication or procedure. The 1-3 scale, when connected to meaningful abilities, is a better thermometer for what you're able to do today. When my pain crossed to level 3 my psychologist repeated the same mantra: "You won't always be here." Over and over she'd say it, reminding me of my days with less pain. We have a wandering intensity, character and even location of pain. My cycle trends towards good weeks and bad weeks. Does your pain fluctuate hourly, weekly or monthly? No matter which, remember:

You won't always be here.

Collecting the Evidence

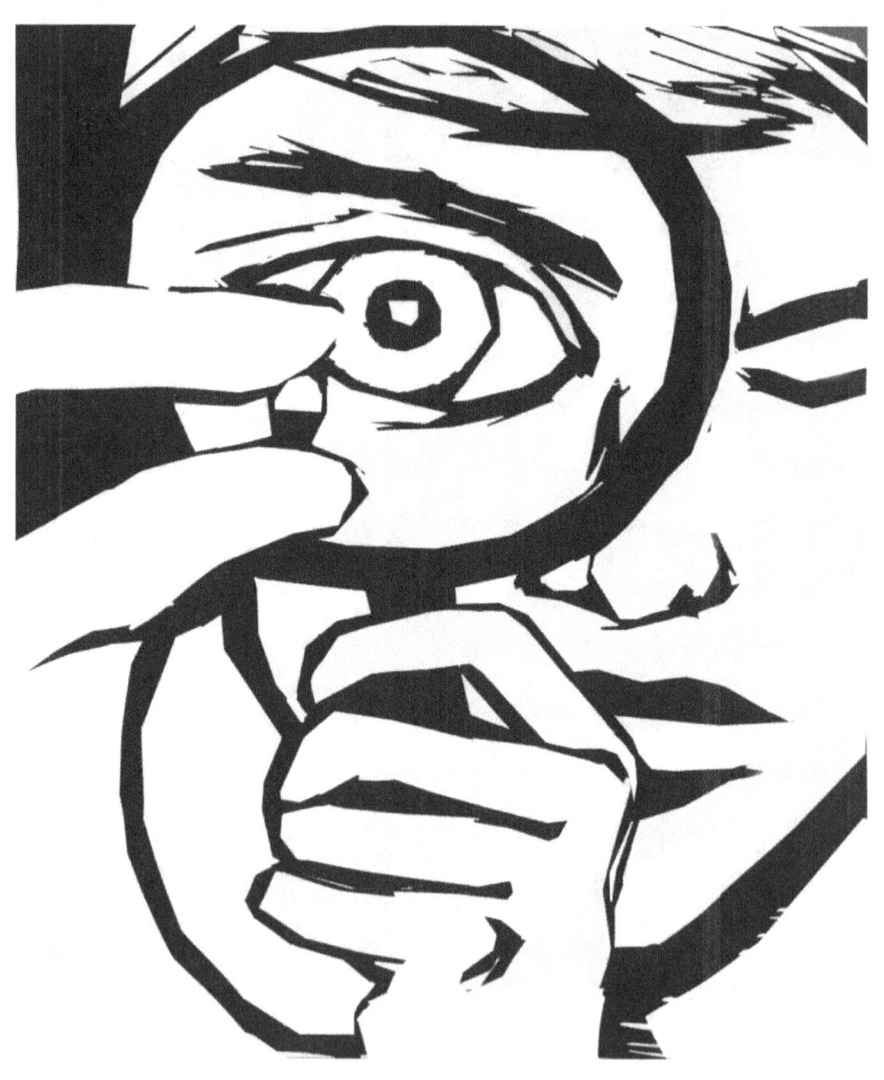

I injured myself playing tennis but developed years of neuropathic pain. It didn't fit. I had pain out of proportion to the type of injury, refused opioid pain killers and continued working. But working with pain was horrible. There was no chit-chat with patients before surgery and no banter with surgeons as they operated. I was curt and rude as every movement fanned the fire of my pain. As I anesthetized patients my groin, buttocks, and hips were front and center in my mind instead of blood pressure, heart rate and oxygen saturation.

During one overnight call a patient was rushed to the operating room with gunshot wounds to the chest. The surgeon tried to twist off the nozzle of the fire hydrant, blood everywhere. And I? One hand transfusing blood back into the patient while the other held an ice pack against my hip. Another memorable day I was doing obstetric anesthesia and argued with a patient over her desire for an epidural. "Women have given birth for centuries without epidurals," I said, in too much pain to perform the procedure.

I soon passed out in the operating room from pain. I was rolling to the ER in a gurney, and remember looking at the fluorescent ceiling lights passing overhead. I looked down at myself and didn't recognize who I saw. The pain had altered my identity, turning me into someone else. I went into medicine to help people, and into anesthesia to soothe nerves before surgery. In that gurney I no longer saw a doctor. I saw a patient.

The Four Pieces of Evidence

I stopped anesthetizing patients to save them from myself. Without work, I turned my attention to rooting out the cause of my pain. The curtain was pulled back and I became the examined, instead of the examiner.

A lawyer gives more credence to physical evidence over witness testimony, so too a doctor begins his search with the provable evidence of pain: X-rays, CT scans and MRIs. "Testimony," the story of the pain's onset, intensity and duration comes last. Expect this. Don't take offense when the doctor turns his back and studies the x-ray. Scans take priority over a patient's history, as DNA takes precedence over eye-witness testimony.

Pain's evidence comes in four varieties, listed in increasing order of importance.

- Intensity—how badly it hurts.
- Character—what kind of pain?
- Precipitating factors—the story of its onset.
- Imaging studies—X-rays, CT scans and MRIs.

I leave out physical exam because it is being replaced by technology in our country. Lungs will be x-rayed, a heart will have an echocardiogram and a knee an MRI. You will get a cursory physical exam, which will serve as an adjunct to the four elements listed above.

If all goes well each piece of evidence will correlate tidily on a yellow brick road to a diagnosis. Voilà! But with chronic pain these four factors will contradict, like a sign-post at a four-way stop. Do you take the road pointed down by the CT scan (a herniated disc), or follow the path of the pain's character (a muscular problem)? Understanding how each piece of evidence aids in the diagnoses will help tilt the compass towards true north.

Intensity

Intensity is rated on a scale from 1 to 10, and measures of how badly it hurts. There is no right or wrong answer to this question. Repeat: There is no right or wrong answer. Your responses are only compared to your previous answers to determine if your pain improves or worsens after a procedure or medication change.

One patient described his back pain as "excruciating," but chose 5 on the 1-10 scale. He was stoic, and his 5 correlated with "horrible and unbearable." He did not need to tell us 10 to convince us of his pain, because he was sitting in a chronic pain clinic. After a steroid injection, he rerated his pain a 2, pleased with the improvement.

Exaggerate your pain, rate it a 13 on a scale from 1 to 10, and you will be taken less seriously. The doctor's initial impression is crucial, because in the age of electronic record-keeping, the way you are defined by one doctor will be visible to all. You don't want to get labeled an exaggerator, drug seeker or head case. Be appropriate, serious and descriptive. Attorneys look for changes in a witness's testimony to impeach them—changes in your pain story will discredit you.

While magnifying pain severity leads to suspicion, exaggerating pain relief causes even greater problems. Reporting pain relief after a procedure if none was achieved, maybe to please your doctor, will lead to further procedures down an incorrect diagnostic line.

In summary, the intensity of pain is not used to diagnose, but to follow progression.

Character

After each appointment your doctor dictates an encounter note which goes into your chart, but will not be forwarded to you. Call record keeping and request them, because they contain your physician's thoughts. You will see some of the following terms describing you pain's character:

- Neuropathic pain: nerve pain.
- Visceral pain: pain from inside abdominal organs.
- Somatic pain: pain from skin, bone or muscle.
- Phantom limb pain: persistent pain from an amputated limb.
- Hyperalgesia: extreme sensitivity to pain.
- Allodynia: an exaggerated response to non-painful events.

Neuropathic pain burns and shoots like lightning, or is dull and continuous. Use the word "burning" and your physician will consider a herniated disc, an entrapped nerve or something else nerve-related (see, you are being categorized).

Visceral pain is from an organ inside your abdomen. There is a scarcity of nerve endings inside the body (most are in the skin), so this pain is vague in location. Intestinal obstruction, a bleeding ulcer or appendicitis present in this manner. Somatic pain is musculoskeletal in origin: a bruised muscle or bone from a fall or injury.

The way you describe your pain gives clue to its cause. Burning pain goes into the nerve pain box, and musculoskeletal pain the somatic pain box. One well-known pain character is kidney stones, which cause agony with minimal pressure to the abdomen, or a shake of the hospital bed. One doctor I knew gave his bed-shake-exam more credence than CT scans when diagnosing kidney stones, a rare example of pain's character trumping imaging studies.

The description of your pain's character is the first decision point in the algorithm (the few that exist for pain), and will slot you into the somatic, visceral or neuropathic pain box. After this initial sorting you're boxed in, and doctors will only consider diagnosis along this branch.

Precipitating Factors

What were you doing before, or when, the pain began? A car crash or fall is obvious, but the injury is often subtle when the pain is chronic. Doctors will try to correlate the mechanism of injury with the severity and character of pain you are experiencing. If they don't correlate, suspicion will be aroused, as happened to me. I was playing tennis, yet developed seven years of burning pain. Tennis injuries lead to somatic pain, muscle or bone, and last for weeks, not years. If I was playing a contact sport, or crushed by a semi, my pain story would have correlated more neatly. I saw raised eyebrows when I described my injury, pain level and duration: "You're taking methadone for a tennis injury?" When you see the raised eyebrow sign, get thee to a pain specialist.

Chronic pain specialists better understand the body's wackiness, such as how a bump can lead to lifelong pain. Family practice doctors and internists don't see these rare cases and will be skeptical (we would be too in their shoes). Besides being less orthodox correlating the injury and severity of pain, pain specialists will be more forgiving of your affect. Have you ever heard, "Well, you don't look like you're in pain?" Give your doctor an Oscar-winning performance with tears and endless diatribes of how the pain has destroyed your life and you'll be labeled "hysterical" or "likely exaggerating." Or enter the pain clinic stoic and soft-spoken, and you'll see written in your chart, "No visible signs of distress." How are we supposed to act when we're hurting? Pain specialists better understand everyone has a different visible response to pain, a different affect.

I discuss this spectrum with my doctors, asking if they'd prefer me on the stoic or hysterical end. This gets me a smile, educates the doctor of the disparate reactions to pain and immediately builds trust.

Imaging Studies

The most important evidence is the imaging studies, because this will try to correlate a visible radiologic abnormality with the pattern of pain described. In my case, CTs and MRIs of my brain, chest, abdomen and pelvis were normal. But I had hair loss and swollen lines of skin wrapping around my pelvis, which is typical for neuropathic pain, and was objective evidence for my doctor to hang his hat on.

Convincing a doctor you have back pain with a normal MRI is akin to convincing a judge you were not at a crime scene when you have no alibi. Both are an absence of evidence, which shouldn't be used as evidence you are lying. But it is. People are people, and an absence of evidence in our society isn't seen as neutral, but evidence against you to overcome. Prevail over this unfairness by being consistent, compliant with instructions and informed.

Chronic pain patients have negative, or confounding, imaging studies, taking away their DNA evidence. As the doctors hunt for more evidence, if only to overcome the guilt associated by a lack of evidence, you will be pushed into some of the following machines.

X-rays: Quick, cheap and safe. A x-ray will precede any MRI or CT scan. It's a quick snapshot of your body, and so has minimal radiation exposure. An x-ray run continuously is called fluoroscopy and is used as guidance during procedures. X-ray's don't show detail as well as MRI and CT scans.

CT or CAT scans: These are super x-rays, last a few seconds, and expose you to more radiation. A chronic pain patient will have many CT scans, because they are cheaper than MRIs ($500 versus $5,000). This is the scan to hunt blindly around your body for the pain generator. CT scans better visualize bone than MRIs.

MRI: This machine uses magnets, not radiation, removing any cancer risk. MRIs are best at visualizing soft tissue, and so are preferred to visualize muscles, ligaments and cartilage (a knee will undergo a MRI, not a CT scan). The downside is the high price tag, time-consumption and claustrophobia-inducing tube.

MRIs are also used as guidance during procedures instead of fluoroscopy. But beware of the practitioner who solely use MRIs and not fluoroscopy for procedures; they do it for the increased reimbursement of the more expensive scan, not the "better image," as you'll be told.

After years of CTs and MRIs, I started refusing them because each scan yielded diminishing returns. As Einstein said, insanity is doing the same thing over and over and expecting different results. How many scans does the same spine need?

Ultrasound: Cheap, quick and safe, ultrasound uses sound waves like a submarine's sonar to penetrate hollow structures—the gallbladder, uterus, arteries and veins—and record the returning reflections.

Arthrogram: The prefix arthro means joint, and the suffix gram means something written or shown (like telegram), so an arthrogram is the "showing of a joint." Contrast (a liquid seen well on x-rays) is injected into a joint, say the knee, and then an x-ray or MRI is taken to better see the inside of the knee.

Laparoscopy: Whenever a camera is put inside the body, the suffix -oscopy is used. Cameras carry no risk of radiation, but require sedation, if not general anesthesia, which does entail risk. Laparoscopy is a camera inserted into the abdomen to evaluate abdominal pain, and endoscopy or colonoscopy is when a camera probes your small intestine or colon to investigate for cancer or other cause of abdominal pain. Arthroscopy is when a camera is put into a joint, the shoulder or knee, to look for damaged cartilage causing pain.

Nerve conduction study (NCS) and Electromyelogram (EMG): These are done together, and is a painful procedure where needles are placed into nerves and muscles, and electricity is sent through them so the speed of the signal, and thus the nerve, can be recorded. You can't be sedated for this because anesthetics interfere with the results. This is a common procedure for pain patients, and is used to rule out rare neurological or muscular diagnoses (Lou-Gehrig's disease, muscular dystrophy or Guillaine-Barre syndrome), but never rules in any diagnosis. You must have this procedure (sorry) to rule out the obscure, even though it won't provide a diagnosis.

Becoming a Detective

Between procedures, test days, waiting for results and doctor appointments, you and I must simply face the pain. Use this time to observe your pain and learn its peculiarities: what triggers and alleviates it?

Here's an example from my life of time well spent. I noticed while walking around the block that as I'd pass in front of a house my groin pain worsened, but standing between houses my pain disappeared. How peculiar. I tested it repeatedly, and got the same result. Where I stood in relation to a house affected my pain.

Walking in a section of town without sidewalks didn't cause pain, so I deduced the sidewalk, and not the house, was responsible. Then it struck me. The slant of the driveway was the difference. Walking across a driveway caused one leg to walk on higher ground, shifting one hip higher and misaligning my pelvis (because the ligaments meant to hold it in place were torn). This led to abnormal movement of the sacroiliac joint (SI joint), which contains nerves traveling into the groin (I'm still impressed I figured this out).

I took this knowledge, how sensitive my pelvis was to misalignment, and investigated other movements causing similar misalignment. Separating my legs in any direction increased my pain, so I shortened my stride. Sleeping on my side hurt, so I put two pillows between my legs to align my pelvis as I slept. Painstakingly (pun intended), every movement was categorized: soft couches hurt, while firm chairs helped; bending at my waist hurt, but bending with my knees didn't; getting out of a car one leg at a time hurt, but twisting my torso as one unit didn't; carrying more than a gallon of milk hurt and anything from the Relax-the-Back store helped.

Deductive reasoning, à la Sherlock Holmes, is the focus on minute detail to divine the cause of something. Employ Holmesian deduction to your day and discover your pain triggers. The modern-day Sherlock Holmes is Dr. Gregory House, or just "House," from the TV show of the same name. He suffers chronic leg pain, a sub-plot of each episode, which covers the dilemmas pain patients encounter each day. He has trouble getting Vicodin prescriptions, suffers withdrawal, argues with physicians and continually searches for a cure. But I bring him up for another point: his perception. He focuses on the details of his patients, clues overlooked by his fellow doctors, to diagnose them correctly. He is the modern-day Sherlock Holmes, even down to the cocaine/Vicodin abuse. Imitate his perception.

Removing ten inappreciably small irritants to your pain, in aggregate, will cause noticeable improvement.

Become a detective and collect your own evidence.

The Chronic Pain Syndrome

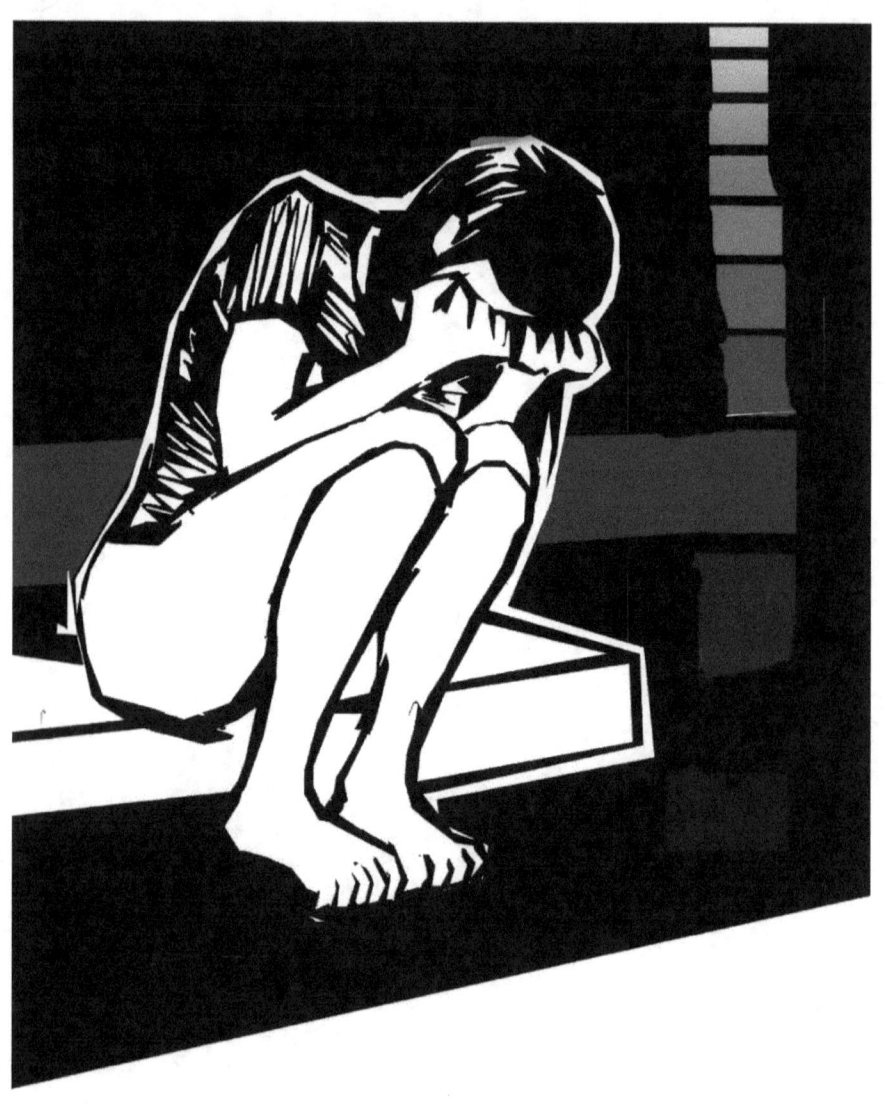

Chronic pain is unrelenting, like ivy. Its stalk extends into all facets of life: social, psychological, financial, work and home. These secondary vines take root and a life of their own. Severing the original stalk and uprooting its underground network doesn't prevent the tenacity of this weed, as curing chronic pain does not wipe out the add-on diagnoses it fathers.

These diagnoses are so common that, in the world of syndromology, they warrant their own name: Chronic Pain Syndrome (CPS henceforth). Pain doctors treat the components of CPS before they even exist, the benefit of prevention so outweighs the risk of side effects. Chronic Pain Syndrome includes:

- Depression
- Anxiety
- Substance abuse
- Catastrophizing
- Guarding
- Negative filtering

- Disability claims
- Sleep disturbance
- Opioid dependence
- Personality disorders
- Social withdrawal/isolation
- Multiple failed surgeries

CPS can cut in line and became the principal diagnosis even after the precipitating cause is diagnosed and cured. Examples include the opioid-dependent patient who crushes and injects her pills, the anxiety-ridden patient unable to leave her house or the depressed patient with suicide attempts. In each the primary diagnosis is chronic pain, but the more troubling opioid dependence, anxiety and depression rise to be the more pressing concern. As the offshoots outgrow the parent, you enter chicken and egg territory, which adds confusion to a thickening medical chart.

Pain patients have a special bipolarity with depression (the downer) and anxiety (the upper) being the two most common diagnoses stemming from chronic pain. A chronic pain patient in the ER with abdominal pain can have depression or anxiety, because both can present this way. Is the anxiety from poorly treated pain? or is the pain controlled and the anxiety rearing its head from the tumult of everyday life? Is the patient depressed because of worsening pain, or just depressed? This patient may leave the ER with medications for pain, anxiety or depression.

You must understand how your body reacts to pain, anxiety and depression to avoid this confusion. Do this by studying how other people's bodies have reacted under similar duress. CPS is a collection of recorded symptoms from past pain patients. I will scratch the surface of 4 of its common components: anxiety, depression, catastrophizing and guarding.

The Pain-Anxiety Response

Pain is ingrained in our genes to cause anxiety, and the explanation is elegant and satisfying. First we need to return to prehistoric times, to the point pain and anxiety were bonded together within our DNA.

Visualize a caveman confronting a tiger in the jungle. A battle begins and the cavemen whose skin is punctured and feels pain will fight harder (and survive) or flee faster (and survive). The caveman who loses an arm and takes time to ponder—that's interesting—will die. Pain was chosen through Darwinian evolution to promote survival. But pain is only the alert system; the response system initiating faster fleeing and better battling is the fight or flight response, sympathetic response or pain-anxiety response.

Injured and in pain, the caveman's body transforms itself to its optimal fighting and fleeing state. The signs (measurable) are an increase in blood pressure, heart rate, breathing rate, sweating, trembling, pupil dilation and pale skin. The blood changes too: fat is broken down to glucose to feed the muscles, and the arteries and veins divert blood away from the intestines towards the muscles. Digestion comes to a halt and we lose peripheral vision (and men lose the ability to get an erection). The symptoms (felt, but not measurable) are restlessness, jumpiness, nervousness and irritability. This is the fight or flight, or pain-anxiety response.

For completeness sake the opposite response is called rest and digest (or parasympathetic response). Everything I mentioned happens in reverse: blood is pumped to the stomach and away from the muscles, pupils constrict, blood glucose drops, heart rate and breathing slow (erections return etc). It kicks in when we are safe in our cave, with the tiger roasting on a spit. We must admire the beauty of the human body.

So cavemen with a nervous system of pain connected to the fight or flight response were chosen by evolution for survival. Anxiety is a natural response to pain. Cut yourself and your blood pressure and heart rate will rise, breathing will quicken and blood glucose levels elevate. As generations pass, Darwin's laws are followed, and this response evolves to initiate not only to pain, but to the threat of pain—the appearance of a predator. If you see a T. Rex your heart rate and blood pressure increase; why wait to get clawed first?

But seeing a tiger in a forest, and seeing a tiger behind a fence in a zoo, don't cause the same response. We know the fence is protecting us from danger at the zoo, so our mind overrides the natural inclination to become anxious; we may even be resting and digesting an ice cream cone while observing the tiger. When you see a caged tiger you know you are safe; so convince yourself you are safe despite pain and you will not experience anxiety. To do this you must become comfortable with your pain. The link between pain and anxiety is fear and the unknown. So making the unknown, known, takes away both the fear and anxiety. Do this by learning the boundaries and intricacies of your pain: What provokes it? How long does it last after each trigger? How assuredly does it go away? This focuses more on preventing the anxiety response, which I discuss in the chapter "Down the Rabbit Hole." But let me stick to treating the pain-anxiety response once it has begun.

Treating Anxiety

Instinctively we know anxiety is bad for us: it's wrecking our bodies from the inside out as we rev up for a fight or flight, with no tiger to battle or run from. So we sit, ready to ride into battle, with a rapid heart rate, sweaty palms and tension. The signs and symptoms of anxiety will be specific to each of us; my anxiety presents as chest pain, and for others it will be shortness of breath, abdominal pain or headaches. Anxiety begins in a millisecond, departs just as fast and is triggered by conscious or unconscious thoughts, sights, sounds or smells. We pain lot are prone to anxiety because we have much worry and uncertainty in our lives. We stand on shaky ground, with the ups and downs of doctor appointments, procedures, new medications, pain flairs and fear of re-injury. We live on a fault line, with continual aftershocks and the occasional large trembler.

Anxiety has its sub-categories, if you want to label your triggers: panic disorder, agoraphobia, specific phobia, social phobia, post-traumatic stress disorder, obsessive compulsive disorder and generalized anxiety disorder. But treatment is all the same.

My first line treatment is positive filtering and distraction. I filter out negative outcomes, focusing on the positive; or I distract myself with a focused task, like fixing something that's broken, watching engaging movies (especially with subtitles), calling a friend to get lost in their world or anything involving instructions (IKEA furniture). The objective is to get the mind, conscious and unconscious, processing information not anxiety related.

Second, I treat it with a brisk walk. Your body is primed for a fight or flight, so use this energy instead of repressing it. This will releases endorphins into the bloodstream causing euphoria (taken to extreme it's called a runner's high).

Third, I turn to the medicine cabinet for the two mainstay treatments: benzodiazepines and beta-blockers. Benzodiazepines are tranquilizers— Valium, Xanax, Ativan, clonazepam, lorazepam—that differ in how long they last. They are habit forming and require a prescription, making doctors wary of prescribing them. But pain specialists, knowledgeable of CPS, will be more liberal. The second medication, beta-blockers, slow the heart rate and stop the hands from trembling (they are prescribed to treat stage fright). Both of these medications produce an anti-fight-or-flight effect (so don't take either if a tiger *is* in front of you).

The third class of medication is the anti-depressant, which also has anti-anxiety properties and prevents the onset of anxiety, but does not treat acute anxiety. Pain specialists begin their patients on anti-depressants as a "weed killer" to prevent the two stalks of anxiety and depression from ever growing.

Pain causes anxiety, but what effect does anxiety have on pain? One study had patients with back pain[7] have electrodes inserted into their back muscles along with a control group without back pain. During a provoked stressful situation, the muscles of the pain group contracted more than the control group, worsening their pain. The take-home message is pain causes anxiety, and anxiety causes pain, creating a positive feedback loop.

Mindfulness of symptoms allows the translation of anxiety's cryptic language into comprehensible words, decreasing its two main engines: fear and the unknown.

Depression

A 2010 study[8] put the prevalence of depression in the chronic pain population at 80% (counting major depression, minor depression and dysthymia). Chronic pain increases the duration of depression by 7 months as well as the severity of depression,[9] and chronic pain is the best predictor of developing depression.[10] Depression is worse if the cause of the chronic pain is unknown.

Symptoms of depression are also symptoms of chronic pain, so differentiating the two is difficult.[11] The most widely used depression scale[12] screens for the following symptoms of depression: depressed mood, guilt, suicidal thoughts, insomnia, agitation, altered thought or speech, anxiety, loss of libido, loss of energy, weight loss, decreased appetite and pain in the back, head, muscles or limbs.

Treating depression in a chronic pain population results in benefits beyond just the depressive symptoms, including a decrease in pain scores, improved function status and better quality of life.[13]

Pain and depression research[14] found other associations: 1) pain is as strongly associated with depression as with anxiety; 2) the pain characteristic most associated with depression is diffuseness of pain; and 3) certain symptoms of depression (low energy, disturbed sleep and worry) are more associated with pain than other depression symptoms (guilt or loneliness). Depression has its sub-categories: major depression, dysthymia, anhedonia, bipolar depression, psychotic depression, catatonic depression, atypical depression. But I prefer my parents' term for anything psychiatric: "not-quite-right."

I was unhappy living in pain, but resisted anti-depressants for years using the excuse depression is a chemical imbalance in the brain of dopamine and serotonin, and what I was experiencing was "appropriate unhappiness." Who wouldn't be depressed in my situation? We wouldn't prescribe anti-depressants for a grieving widow; psychiatrists argue the grieving process is therapeutic and necessary to accepting such a loss. So why is grieving the loss of my former life any different? But the most recent version of psychiatric diagnosis, the DSM-V, did consider adding bereavement as a medical condition,[15] until an uproar changed their minds.

But one day I had an aha moment, changing my opinion. I was experiencing minimal pain and walking along the riverfront listening to NPR podcasts. Yet walking besides me was an uninvited companion, unhappiness. Psychiatrists call it anhedonia, a state below depression defined as a persistent lack of joy, but I recognized it as not-quite-right. Alcoholics describe their moment of clarity, and this was mine. Why wasn't I happy during this moment of painlessness? I was the widower whose wife had been resurrected, yet continued grieving.

I sought help. I started on an anti-depressant, changed to a second, and progressed down the list of those best suited for pain patients. I had side effects from the SSRIs, the most commonly prescribed anti-depressants, and the most advertised anti-depressant for pain patients, Cymbalta, did nothing for my mood after a trial of multiple months. But the third drug I tried, bupropion (Wellbutrin), lifted a veil I didn't know existed. It had zero effect on my pain, but an impressive impact on my mood; I had energy in the morning, felt like doing things in the day, and was...chipper.

My experience was unusual in how quickly the medication worked, as there is evidence pain patients need to be titrated to high doses over weeks to obtain an impact on their mood and pain. I still had pain and anxiety, but the vine of depression (whichever subcategory) was gone. One yellow pill every morning removed the blinders darkening my world.

Depression Treatment

Anti-depressants don't work.

Well, let me be more specific. Anti-depressants aren't any better than placebo for mild, moderate or severe depression. Anti-depressants do work better than placebo for very severe depression.

But what about my yellow pill, and the blinders being removed? Well, I like the color of my pill, and its size and shape, which all add to its placebo effect. But the evidence is clear, it doesn't perform any better than a tic-tac, so long as the label is changed from tic-tac to anti-depressant.

I first heard about this from a *60 Minutes* segment[16] in 2012, then found a 2010 meta-analysis[17] in JAMA with data from pooled RCTs (Randomized Controlled Trials) concluding the benefits of anti-depressants "were nonexistent to negligible among depressed patients with mild, moderate, and even severe baseline symptoms, whereas they were large for patients with very severe symptoms."

The gold-standard depression screening categories are: 0-7=normal; 8-13 = mild depression; 14-18 = moderate depression; 19-22 = severe depression and 23 or greater = very severe depression. Anti-depressants were clinically superior to placebo at depression scores of 25 or greater. For depression less than 25 they did not reach statistical significance over placebo.

But before you dump your anti-depressants down the toilet, there's a distinction to make. This study, and the one discussed on the *60 Minutes* segment, is not saying anti-depressants don't work; rather, they do work, and so do placebos. The placebo effect is powerful and real, as I'll discuss later. The chemicals in anti-depressant tablets should be reserved for the depressed patient that's catatonic; and the sugar for the rest of us.

The take-home is this: anti-depressants do help depression via the placebo effect. Do you really care *how* they work? I don't.

Catastrophizing

Catastrophic is a fitting word to describe our pain. Too fitting, it turns out. The adjective was pulled from our lexicon, transformed by physicians into a verb, and offered back to us as yet another label to diagnose us with. So what is catastrophizing?

It's broadly defined as an exaggerated negative mental mindset in response to actual or anticipated pain and is subdivided (ahem) into magnification (the exaggeration of symptoms), helplessness (feeling powerless), pessimism (expecting bad outcomes) and rumination (obsessively mulling negative events).

Like everything, when done in proportion it's appropriate; but done too much it's pathologic. Excess woe leads to a death spiral causing more pain intensity, disability and psychological distress.[18]

Catastrophizing predicts future pain severity[19] and physical impairment.[20] Patients in a pain-free state were evaluated on a written catastrophe scale, and these scores predicted their pain scores in response to painful stimuli weeks later.[21] Catastrophe scores of arthritis patients predicted their pain upon return to the clinic six months later.[22] Catastrophizing is associated with increased medication use,[23] suicidal ideation,[24] illness behavior,[25] hospitalizations[26] and clinic visits.[27] And because pain-related disability accounts for enormous lost productivity, these studies were well-funded. The consensus is: "catastrophizing has been associated with heightened disability, even when controlling for depression, anxiety, neuroticism, disease severity, and pain severity."[28]

What can we do? Is catastrophizing a part of our personality, or does the admonition "stop sniveling" decrease catastrophizing, and ultimately pain? The answers are yes, and yes. Our catastrophe level remains relatively constant throughout life, but psychological intervention decreases pain intensity, disability and psychological distress[29] by impartially evaluating, and defusing the created doomsday scenario. If based on an incorrect belief, the cascading consequences of catastrophizing end in utter calamity:

I can't work because of pain	→	I'll have no income	→	I'll lose my house	→	my spouse will leave me

I experienced this effect firsthand on my catastrophic days ($^{10}/_{10}$ pain). I'd run to my psychologist feeling helpless, and she'd talk me down by repeating her mantra, "You won't always be here." Once settled, she'd get tough, telling me to snap out of it and stop exaggerating. She defused me, and I left her office feeling better than when I went in.

Guarding

If you're the type of person who enjoys people watching, the most fascinating place to do this is in the waiting room of a pain clinic (yes, even more so than the airport). Patients wear their hearts on their sleeves; every sign and symptom of CPS will be visible over a half hour's time. Near-empty pill bottles clutched tightly by those entering the clinic are transformed into prescription-toting patients, with a spring in their step, making a beeline for the door (and pharmacy). Sleep deprivation, anxiety and depression meld on the countenances of the patients' faces, forming a strange, disheartened look. Silence hangs in the air as everyone keeps to themselves, holding disability forms, x-rays, canes and wheelchair arms. No one verbally complains of pain because there's no one listening, but the non-verbal pain behaviors are easy to spot.

These pain behaviors are lumped into the category guarding: "any behavior that prevents or reduces pain. Guarding behavior includes stiffness, limping, bracing a body part and flinching."[30] Back pain patients ease themselves into a chair, supporting themselves on the arms of the chair as long as possible. Patients with extremity pain will have an invisible force field around their painful appendage; enter this field of space and they'll growl, "Back off." Spinal fusion patients are so afraid of wrecking their newly fused spines they walk on eggshells. It's a natural instinct to be protective of our bodies in pain; but the pain patient takes it to a whole new level. Movement restriction for too long becomes second nature and leads to muscular de-conditioning and worsening pain.

A group of patients with back pain was followed and studied at intervals using tests of fitness, pain level, disability level, guarding, mental health and reintegration into the workforce. Patients who exhibited guarding were the least likely to return to work, and if they did return, the most likely to have the most absentee days. Guarding is the best predictive factor of who will and who won't return to work, which suggests a transition has been made from acute to chronic pain.[31] This is a perfect time for a radical intervention, before the routine becomes reflex.

I remember the incredulous look on my surgeon's face as I un-cinched and removed the lumbar back brace I had been wearing for two years after my second spinal fusion. "I recommend patients wear this brace for six weeks," he said. "Any longer and your muscles will shrivel."

"Oh," I replied, keeping an eagle eye on the brace and away from his clutching talons. I was displaying guarding behavior, babying and protecting my back from every bump. I curtailed my physical therapy, pointing to my back brace as an excuse. This obsession of protecting my back added to my social isolation ("I must stay home and lie flat"), depression ("I have no friends"), anxiety ("My back!") and substance abuse ("There's nothing else to do but drink").

"I still feel movement in my back," I told my doctor, his eyes betraying a flicker of suspicion. But a complaint carries a lot more weight with an M.D. behind it, so he let me cinch up the brace again. What I didn't realize was my guarding behavior, one of the best predictors of the transition from acute to chronic pain, was another checkmark in front of the long list of CPS symptoms I was accumulating.

A Diagnosis Unto Itself

Consider hip pain. A *primary* cause is osteoarthritis; the *secondary* diagnosis is again chronic pain; and *tertiary* irritants would be going up stairs, financial insecurity or even a pitying spouse (attention to pain worsens it[32]). Each should be treated as a stand-alone diagnosis. The primary osteoarthritis will improve with steroid shots or a hip replacement. The secondary chronic pain needs "winding down" with ice, NSAIDS or anti-convulsant medications (these stop abnormal nerve firing, a hallmark of both seizures and chronic pain). And the tertiary environment needs optimizing: time off work, ergonomic changes, psychological counseling and a supportive doctor-patient relationship. Fear and anxiety lower the pain threshold and increase sensitivity to pain (*hyperalgesia* and *allodynia*)[33]; this is why there is rarely a link between injury severity, x-ray findings and pain level.[34]

But chronic pain will not be cracked until the human brain is unraveled. A decade long Brain Activity Map[35] is being considered, now the Human Genome Project is finished. But let's put this project in perspective. Mapping the one *million* neurons in the brain of a mouse would create equivalent data as the Hadron Collider in Geneva, which smashes atoms together to analyze the debris. The human brain has 85 to 100 *billion* neurons, a 300,000 times larger undertaking, dwarfing the Manhattan Project, man on the moon or any other contemporary venture. A better analogy is the multi-generational construction of the Egyptian pyramids. Some pharaoh had to have the foresight to cut that first cornerstone, knowing he'd never live to see the capstone in place. Such is the enormity of mapping the brain, and understanding chronic pain

Treating Chronic Pain Syndrome

As pain invades your life, treatment needs to take its omnipresence into consideration. Treating the pain alone will leave a depressed, anxious, substance-abusing patient who overly guards and catastrophizes. The biopsychosocial model of pain management advocates treating each invaded area: biological, psychological and social.

Medicine is full of cause and effect examples. Lung cancer leads to pneumonia; high cholesterol to heart attack; chemotherapy to infection; AIDS to fungal pneumonia and colon cancer to anemia. Doctors screen for these common associated diagnoses; but this is more difficult with chronic pain because more organ systems are affected: the mind, heart, lungs, muscles and nerves. A pain specialist will (should) screen for each element of CPS at every appointment, treating new symptoms early and fiercely.

Which diagnosis of Chronic Pain Syndrome do you have?

The Pain-Prone Patient

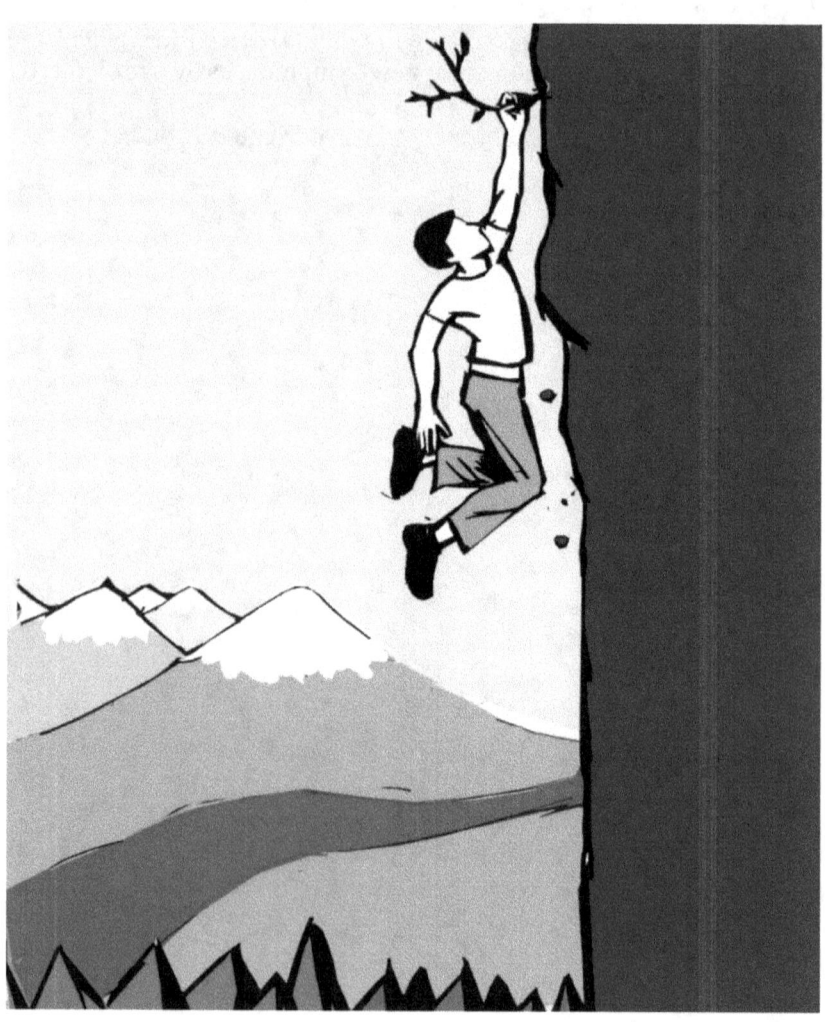

"Even though [patients] complain of pain, for them the pain is almost a comfort or an old friend.... It is an adjustment, a way of adaptation..."

—*Psychogenic Pain*[36]

"Have you ever considered the pain is all in your head?"

Pose this to a pain patient and you'll get her blood up, and a tongue-lashing: "Oh, so I'm faking it?" or, "Do you think I'm having these surgeries for fun?" I was asked this question after six years of pain, and I answered similarly. But the question lingered: Are all pain patients asked this question? We acquire new sickness from Chronic Pain Syndrome,[37] but after the pain has begun, a fruit of the pain. But are we different before the pain begins? Does something predispose us to develop pain, the way black men are susceptible to high blood pressure, or high cholesterol leads to heart disease?

One study[38] dipped its toe in this water, evaluating how a physical trauma—circumcision—affects the pain response half a year later. Circumcised infants cry longer after vaccination than non-circumcised infants, and topical anesthesia given before circumcision decreases this pain response. If the physical trauma of circumcision affects the "pain experience" half a year later, does circumcision make men more aggressive, prone to fighting, injury, disability, suicide and incarceration than women?[39] That's a leap! But a study[40] has identified traits—insults—present before the onset of chronic pain, not nearly as common in non-pain patients:

- Having verbally or physically abusive parents.
- Physical or sexual abuse as a child.
- Having a parent with illness or pain.
- Having a parent with pain of the same gender as the patient.
- Having pain in the same location as a parent.
- Disturbances in interpersonal relationships and work life.

"Pain proneness" presumes pain has an emotional component, called psychogenic or psychosomatic pain. These patients do experience pain, and shouldn't be confused with patients who are malingering (truly "faking it"). Psychogenic pain has a partial, or complete, emotional ingredient—a comfort or an old friend—instead of a sole physical aspect. Their pain is in their heads, not their bodies, but they are experiencing pain nonetheless. The updated criteria of psychogenic pain are listed in the endnotes.[41]

Illness Behavior

When we become sick society treats us differently, which affects the way we act. The new conduct is called illness behavior, and is defined as an observable action communicating someone's perception of their disturbed health. An arthritis patient will rub her joints; a back pain patient will ease into a chair with her arms; and a migraine sufferer will rub her temples. They want you to know of their distress, so they show you by playing up the physical aspects—the greater the distress, the more grandiose the behavior. It's not a conscious or knowing behavior, but does have an outsized influence in chronic pain.[42]

Some illness behavior is normal (we all want attention during catastrophe), but disproportionate "acting" is a sign of other stressors.[43] New guarding or catastrophizing in a patient will be a manifestation of the insecurity of losing health insurance, the ending of a relationship or the failure of a procedure. The doctor needs to ask the question: Why is this patient, exhibiting this symptom, at this time?

The Sick Role

Patients with long term illnesses also assume a sick role, with emphasis on the word role, because there is acting involved. The individual and society are both protagonists in a drama, with four acts:[44]

- The sick person can't be blamed for her illness.
- The sick person is exempt from normal duties while sick.
- She must view the illness as undesirable and must get well.
- The patient must seek medical help and cooperate with doctors.

Society fulfills the first two definitions, obliging the patient to fulfill the third and fourth to hold up her end of the bargain. We excuse the worker with a "head cold" from a day of work, and the patient recovering from a heart attack for multiple weeks; but with chronic pain, society's expectation to get well is not met (violating definition three) and leads to strife between patient and doctor (violating definition four). Wanting to maintain the perception of blamelessness and exemption from duties (1 and 2) leads the patient to exaggerate the visible aspects of her illness. I have personal experience with this.

Four back operations put me into a I'm-recovering-from-surgery mindset for half a decade. I walked with two canes for years, then one cane; and finally abandoned the sticks altogether. Each transition coincided with a noticeable change in treatment. With two canes people sprinted to hold doors, load my groceries into my car and pump my gas. No one asked as to my diagnosis (not wanting to hear the ghastliness).

Walking with one cane downgraded my status: people still held doors, when convenient; the grocery bagger hesitated when I asked for help, unsure if I was serious; and everyone inquired how my "recovery" was progressing (assuming I'd had knee surgery, specifically ACL repair).

When I closeted the canes, the demotion was profound: doors were slammed on me; I was shoulder-checked on the street; and heard sighs when asking for help getting a bag into a plane's overhead bin. New York City, wherever I went.

I once put a folding chair in the handicapped section of a cinema, but the manager scolded me because the space was reserved for wheelchairs. I fired back, "I was shot in the spine in Iraq defending this country, and now I can't put a folding chair in a handicapped section?" Lying, I was acting out the sick role, though my props were gone. To maintain my exempt status—"I'm sick"— I stuttered to recover, prolonging my pain.

Female Hysteria

A historical example of the sick role and illness behavior is 19th century female hysteria: its symptoms were fainting, nervousness, insomnia, shortness of breath, irritability and "a tendency to cause trouble."[45] The treatment was manual manipulation of the genitals by a physician until "hysterical paroxysm"—orgasm—which was thought to cure the malady. The fainting couch became a popular piece of home furniture for these weekly house calls, with some women creating entire fainting rooms.

But something odd happened in the 20th century; the disease, which one doctor said affected a quarter of all women, disappeared. Was it cured? No. The sympathy and attention was replaced with suspicion as the public better understood psychological disorders. The behavior originated in the societal response of increased attention, blamelessness and being excused from chores. The patient played her part by manifesting the expected symptoms, completing the loop. But when the pity stopped, the loop was broken, and the illness behavior was no more.

Fluency in the body's language is worthwhile, but obsession with the self leads common sensations to be mistranslated as serious disease.[46] Every belly ache isn't appendicitis, every headache isn't a brain tumor.

Pain Pathways

Pain receptors in the skin send signals along the nervous system to the brain to protect us from harm. External input is required as these tracts are laid down: seeing, hearing, smelling and touching are necessary for development. But once in place, external input is not needed for the brain to perceive the sensations. Schizophrenics and drug users have visual and auditory hallucinations; alcohol withdrawal causes tactile hallucinations (insects crawling on the skin); and epileptics have gustatory hallucinations (tasting foods not present). Similarly, the brain can suffer pain hallucinations—pain without an external source.

The pain pathways develop during childhood, when psychological trauma (neglect, abandonment or abuse) can sensitize the brain to pain, strengthening its link to the periphery. Roads become freeways. If this person then experiences trauma later in life, like the ending of a relationship, her pain pathways are primed, more than in the non-abused person, to transform anxiety into real physical pain: psychogenic pain.

Psychogenic Pain

Pain exists on a spectrum. At one end lives the patient with chiefly emotional pain and a small actual injury, which is best treated with antidepressants and anti-anxiety medications. On the other end dwells the twisted spine from a car wreck, who will respond best to pain medications. But no one is 100% free of emotional insults, so the partial emotional component of all pain deserves attention.

Pure psychogenic pain, the far end of the spectrum, can be diagnosed with a procedure I did once in my training. Our patient complained of pain in the legs, pelvis and stomach and had failed all treatment. The notion of psychogenic pain arose, and we admitted her to the ICU to test the hypothesis. We performed spinal anesthesia on her, numbing her from toes to mid-chest. After ensuring her nerves were blocked by poking her feet with a needle under the sheets, we asked if she still felt her typical pain (areas now insensate). She said she did; agony as usual. She had pure psychogenic pain.

This chapter sprang from the question, "Have you ever considered the pain is all in your head?" I have Chronic Pain Syndrome—anxiety, depression, substance abuse, sleep disturbance—which arose after my pain started, but no harbinger of pain-proneness. Also, a leg length discrepancy from a torn pelvic ligament turned up and was treated. After this my pain level dropped, and persists at this lower level (changing my condition from being predominantly pain-driven, to disability-driven). But I still hurt every day, even though the problem was correctly diagnosed and "fixed." Why?

How Acute Pain Turns Chronic

Acute pain turns chronic when it outlasts its protective function and is pointless. Why acute pain turns chronic is a darned Sudoku puzzle, but how it occurs is understood. Let's use the earlier patient who knocked her elbow on a doorframe, causing pain from shoulder to hand. A series of events progress from the soft tissue, to the nerve, spinal cord, brainstem and brain cortex. First, a "soup" of inflammatory signals (*neurotransmitters*) flow into the soft tissue,[47] bombarding the pain receptors. The nerves are overwhelmed and lose control (*neurogenic inflammation*): blood vessels swell, leak, and the skin becomes red, pale, hot or cold. Over months the hair, nails and bones deform…and of course, there's pain.

Repeatedly cued to transmit, the pain receptors become hyper-sensitive and send signals when not asked (*ectopic discharges*), or multiply a single signal into many (*after-discharges*). The signals travel upstream to the spinal cord, which steps up and enhances its connection to the peripheral nerve (*synaptic strengthening*). The pain is green-lit from skin to spinal cord in a carpool lane. There's a "winding up" of the spinal cord (*central sensitization*), increasing sensitivity to painful stimuli (*hyperalgesia*) and misinterpreting non-painful stimuli as painful (*allodynia*). Onward it goes, the pain, a twister laying waste as it marches on.

The brainstem (*thalamus*) is a switchboard between spinal cord and brain: it receives signals, interprets them and forwards them to the correct lobe of the brain's cortex. Chronic pain increases the brainstem's background activity, abnormal firing and after-discharges.[48] A MRI of the chronic-pain-brain is anatomically different than the acute-pain-brain[49] (this re-molding is called *neuroplasticity*).[50] These changes are permanent and persist after the original trigger is removed.

Brain tissue—the cortex, or meat of the brain—is allocated in proportion to the body part's sensitivity, not size. A hefty chunk is assigned to the fingertips, while only a sliver to the skin of the back.[51] The beleaguered brain increases the allocated cortex covering the painful body part; the slice of the brain covering the elbow becomes larger. It then grabs more body real estate: pain the size of a golf ball expands to the size of a baseball (or softball…or beach ball!).[52]

I tore a pelvic ligament, causing hip pain, then hair loss, redness, heat and swelling. Misdiagnosed, the acute turned chronic, and the pain traveled faster along the nerve, winding up the spinal cord into a tizzy. This buzz was passed to the brainstem, then cortex, which swelled to process all the traffic. The enlarged cortex then expanded its coverage area: pain spread down my groin, around my flank and to my lower back. When I was correctly diagnosed and treated, the brain and nervous system had been remolded, so pain that began as a symptom of another diagnosis, is now the diagnosis.

This is the crux of chronic pain.

Chronic Pain *is* the diagnosis.

Flex the Complex, Break the Brittle

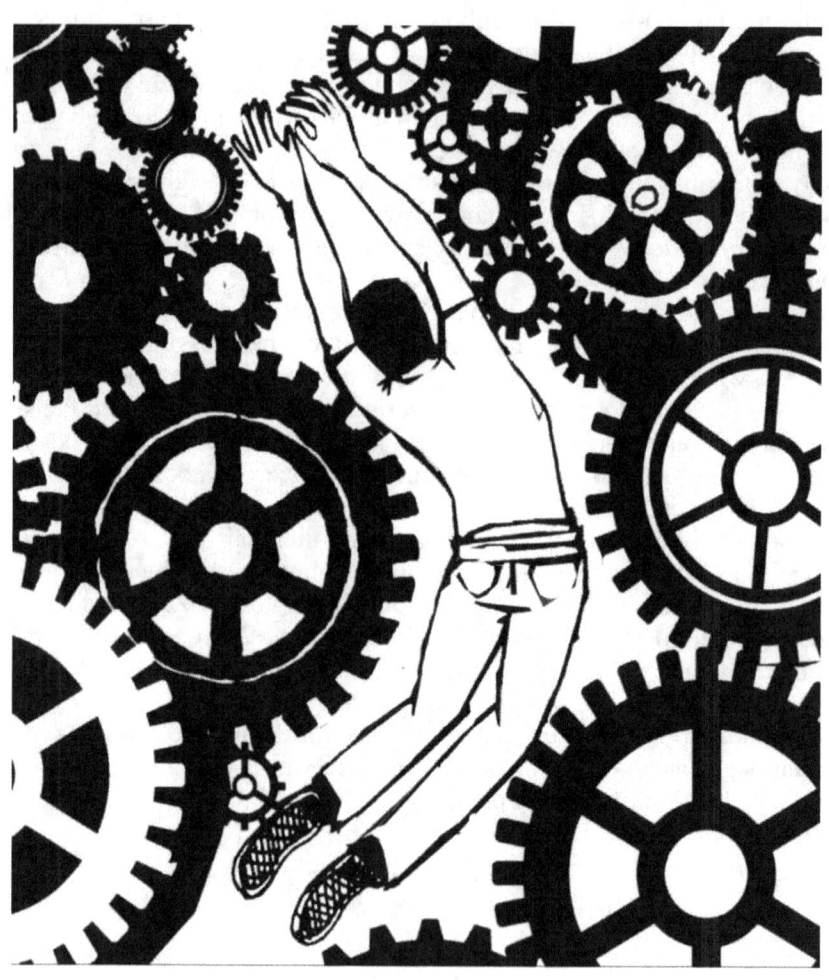

"Even when a system is dissected into its basic parts, those parts are still influenced by a whirligig of forces we can't understand or haven't considered or don't think matter. Hamlet was right: There really are more things in heaven and Earth than are dreamt of in our philosophy."

—*Wired Magazine*

Chronic pain is complex. Treatments must be flexible. Alexander the Great's solution to the Gordian knot—unable to untie it, he sliced through it with his sword—is a model for the treatment of chronic pain: out-of-the-box thinking.

The Three Paradigms of Pain

There have been three paradigms of understanding regarding pain. The first, by René Descartes, likens the body to a machine, and pain to "fast moving particles of fire...[which] pass along the nerve filament until it reaches the brain."[53] This equates tissue damage to pain: the worse the injury, x-ray or scar, the worse the pain. Though twice replaced, this model is ingrained and still affects decisions, as doctors try to cut out the pain generator, or snip the nerves that connect it to the brain. While theoretically sound, this model collapses when carried into the laboratory of life. It doesn't explain why a paper cut sears like a hot brand, but a surfer whose leg becomes lunch for a shark only feels a "bump."[54] If it fails so fantastically—a disarticulated limb is but a knock!—why is it still looked to in pain clinics? Do the planets still revolve around the Earth? Injury severity, x-ray abnormalities and tissue damage *do not* estimate pain severity. Period.

A second model (*gate control theory*) proposes different nerves carry different data: one carries pain, a second touch and a third temperature information. These crowd through a "gate" at the spinal cord, which only allows a set number of signals to pass at once. Traffic jams occur.

A stubbed toe flings open the gate, passes data to the brain, and creates the sensation of pain. The instinct to squeeze a stubbed toe activates the touch and pressure nerves, whose signals pass through the same gate en route to the brain, creating a bottleneck. The squeezing and rubbing purposely clogs the gate with these "other" signals, crowding out the pain signals, decreasing the pain sensation. It's this theory that underpins the functioning of the TENS unit and spinal cord stimulator. And signals going in the other direction, from brain to gate, influence the gates opening and closing, explaining how psychology and the mind affect pain.[55]

So go on, run your own science experiment—snap your finger in a latch; whack your forehead with a cabinet; crack your knee on a coffee table. Now, follow your instinct: rub, squeeze, shake. Jumble the pain signal with these others. Oh elegant science, how you unriddle this sphinx.

Today's Paradigm

Today's paradigm—the *biopsychosocial model*—defines pain as "an unpleasant sensory and emotional experience associated with actual or potential tissue damage." Let's break it down to its three parts: bio/psycho/social. *Bio* unites Descartes' model (tissue damage = pain) with the gate control model (squeeze toe, flood gate). Psycho represents the mind and emotions, which worsen or ease pain. And social take into account the environmental interactions with the patient (*sick role*, *illness behavior* and *pain proneness*). A complex definition for a complex illness. But still it fails to explain the oddities of pain—the needle through the toe that doesn't hurt until noticed and cancer that goes undetected because it's painless.[56] Ongoing studies are probing these areas.

A study compared civilians undergoing surgery to soldiers with equivalent injuries: 32% of the soldiers required opioids compared to 83% of the civilians.[57] You see, for the soldiers their injuries meant an escape from the battlefield, a purple heart and a plane-ticket home. But for civilians surgery is catastrophic. Each group attached a meaning to their pain, which affected their pain experience and morphine requirements. Meaning explains why a finger injury hurts a professional violinist more than an ordinary person.[58] How badly you're hurt doesn't equate with how badly it hurts, and how badly it hurts depends on why it hurts.

Subjects exposed to a painful stimulus rated their pain level to both male and female experimenters chosen for their attractiveness. Male subjects reported less pain in front of female experimenters, and female subjects reported more pain to male experimenters. [59]

Overt pain behavior, guarding, is the best predictor of who will not return to work.[60] Exhibited pain behavior elicits reinforcing responses from society,[61] which increases the pain behavior, augmenting the loop (remember how female hysteria disappeared once the attention stopped). Patients with more doting spouses experience more pain than those with less attentive spouses[62]—attention to pain causes the hurt to hurt more.

These psycho-social aspects of pain continue to surprise investigators, who confirm the impact stress, anxiety, meaning, expectations and exhibited behavior have on the pain experience.

Referred Pain

Let's use examples to illustrate pain's tricky relationship with the mind and environment. A construction worker admitted to the ER with a crushed foot will experience more pain without health insurance than someone fully insured. A bachelor will hurt less than a father with five children to support. In each case, the background meaning affects the pain experience.

The environment also affects the pain felt: imagine the difference being a patient at the Mayo Clinic versus a run-down hospital in Nigeria? The food, the stability of a marriage, visitors and the doctor's appearance and confidence will all affect pain.[63] So what's reliable? It's his foot that's injured, so it'll be his foot that's in pain…right? Not so fast grasshopper, let's turn to referred pain.

Referred pain happens when nerves with high sensory input, like the skin, enter the spinal cord at the same level as nerves with typically low sensory input, like internal organs. The classic example is a heart attack patient with left arm pain, but no chest pain. The dying heart muscle alerts the brain to its peril. But the heart is like the grandson gone off to college; the brain isn't used to hearing from it, so isn't conditioned to respond. The brain is familiar with the skin of the left arm and hand, which tweets all day long like a hungry chick. The nerves from both, heart muscle and arm, enter the spinal cord at the same level. The heart's cry for help is mistaken as arm pain; the brain confuses the two, and a heart attack is *referred* to the left shoulder, arm and hand. Referred pain.

Charts and diagrams illustrate all the patterns of referred pain that have been deciphered. A torn aorta and inflamed pancreas can present as back pain, while inflamed abdominal organs will irritate the diaphragm and present as shoulder pain. Because of referred pain, what hurts is not always what's wrong.

Section 2 carries this complexity into the clinic as physicians try to make diagnoses from varied pain presentations. The diagnosis is crucial: from it stems treatment, and all treatment will fall down in front of a misdiagnosis (changing your oil will not fix a flat tire). A phenomenon in science called error carried forward exists: in a chain of events where one item depends on the next, an upstream error will float downstream leading to a terminal error. Erroneously complain of burning leg pain, when you mean aching leg pain, and your doctor will diagnose neuropathic pain because of the word "burning," implement studies for nerve pain and begin treatment for nerve pain. What happened is you used the wrong adjective to describe your symptoms (muscle pain *aches*, nerve pain *burns*). Language and adjectives matter, and can prevent errors, errors that carry forward.

Flexibility of Treatment

Be flexible and seek flexible physicians (not gymnasts), where open-mindedness exists on both sides. Here's what I mean: I once had an elderly patient with full body pain. Doctors inject lidocaine, local anesthetic, at the site of a patient's pain to numb the pain generator and provide relief. My higher-up decided to give her an intravenous infusion of lidocaine into her blood—"Since she hurts everywhere, let's pump the lidocaine everywhere." It was a novel, and dangerous, approach; intravenous lidocaine risks initiating heart arrhythmias. But after informed consent we began the infusion, and she had an excellent response that lasted for weeks. This is an example of the out-of-the-box thinking valuable in a care provider.

Section one of this book presented experiences you will encounter during your first year of pain: inflammation communicates harm; how physicians approach pain; the doctor-patient relationship; the evidence used in search of a diagnosis; the importance of a correct diagnosis; the co-diagnosis of the chronic pain syndrome; and the complexity and flexibility necessary for confronting pain.

But pain is still poorly understood: getting diagnosed correctly is hit-or-miss; treated correctly, more miss than hit; and obtaining relief often a whiff of the bat. The arbitrary approach of practitioners will demand your adaptability, open-mindedness and perseverance. Flexibility involves being open to novel treatments, while still accepting failure and acknowledging an entire line of attack, your diagnosis, is wrong.

My father once told me, "Find one doctor and stick with him," and the next month, "Keep looking until you find a doctor to diagnose you correctly." As we begin the treatment section, you will feel this same push and pull my father unwittingly expressed.

Battle complexity with flexibility.

II. Treating the Pain

"The body is 'silent,' very quietly performing its functions without compelling moment-to-moment awareness. Only when a foot falls asleep does it attract much attention; only when hunger gnaws are we reminded that there is an internal organ called the stomach. … [T]he chronic pain patient stands in dramatic contrast: He or she is exquisitely and perpetually aware of the body. Within the body is housed the pain, which has become the most salient aspect of daily existence."

—Sandra Thomas,
A Phenomenologic Study of Chronic Pain

First, Do No Harm

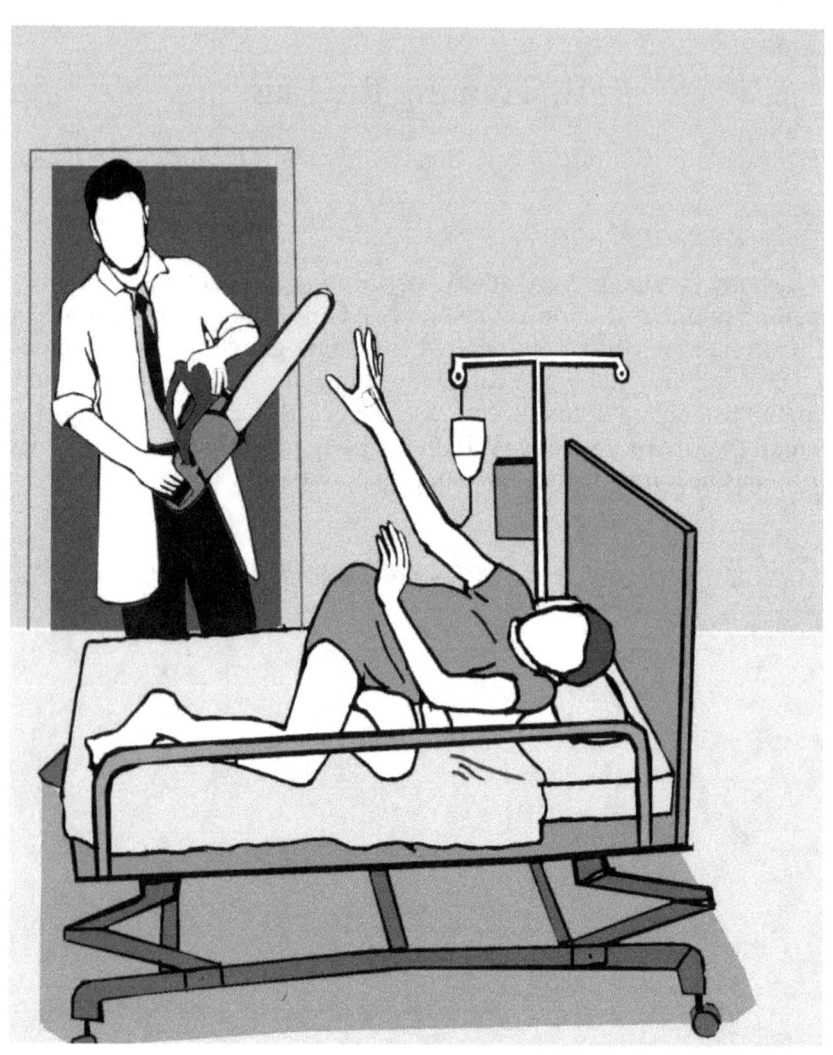

"As to diseases make a habit of two things—to help, or at least, to do no harm."

—Hippocrates

Medicine advances and patients expect treatment on demand—even when the best treatment is no treatment. Before I step us into the pain clinic, I present here two examples of medicine *harming* patients. These are blatant examples that prompt the question: "How can this be?" Yet if this happens when under a national microscope, imagine the harm when the process is not as transparent; when a patient is tucked away in a procedure room without access to evidence, or oversight.

Throughout this chapter keep this one question in mind: If this can happen, then what else...?

The Breast Cancer Debacle

Mammograms cause horrible disfigurement and toxic full-body illness; well, not the exam itself, but the "next step" it leads to. Screening mammograms *do* detect cancer and save lives, but a percentage of women will have cancer detected when there is none (a false positive), leading to a biopsy (and more false positives), and the standard surgery-chemo-radiation regimen. Women without cancer *will* travel to the end of this path; all avoided if their benign mass had only remained hidden. But how to differentiate a lump that will kill from a lump that's just a lump?

A 2009 study[64] revealed screening mammograms reduce breast cancer deaths by 15%, but falsely diagnose women with cancer 30% of the time. For every 2000 women screened over 10 years: 1 will have her life prolonged, 10 will be errantly diagnosed and treated for cancer and 200 will be told they have cancer (and suffer months of psychological distress until it's ruled benign). A statistician put it simpler, "a decade of mammogram screening for a woman in her 40s will increase her lifespan by 5 days, but this will disappear if she rides a bicycle without a helmet for 15 hours (or 50 hours with a helmet)."[65]

Breast cancer risk increases with age: the younger the screened population the more false positives (and errant treatments), while the older the screened population the more false negatives (missed cancers). There is an ideal screening age to minimize both catastrophes—deaths from undetected cancer (*mortality*) and suffering from unnecessary treatments (*morbidity*)—which statisticians determine with graphs, data and powerful computers. A "sweet spot" will emerge—start screening significantly above or below this age and cancer will be under or over detected.

Data from 600,000 women revealed this age was higher than the currently recommended 40, so a panel increased the recommended screening age to 50 (for women with no risk factors).[66] This change minimizes the suffering of women treated for non-existent cancer, and maximizes the number of women correctly diagnosed with cancer. But no screening eradicates all outliers: women with cancer missed, and women mistakenly diagnosed.

Raising the screening age led to a public outcry of Obama's "death squads" and rationing of health care. Surgeons argued screening women in their 40s decreases mortality (which it does, while disproportionally increasing the morbidity of the false positives). The outliers—women in their 40s dying of breast cancer—were trotted out and the more-mammograms-the-better contingency carried the day; Obama backed down and the evening news reported mammogram screening was a "personal decision" for each woman to make.

The evidence is clear for patients without risk factors: *too* early mammogram screening harms more than heals. But emotion trumps mathematics, and the practice continues, harming women they purport to be helping.

If this can happen, then what else…?

The Prostate Cancer Debacle

A more extreme example is the PSA test (prostate specific antigen), which looks for markers in the blood for prostate cancer. The longer a man lives the more likely he is to develop prostate cancer: 10% of men in their 50s and 70% of men in their 80s have prostate cancer.[67] But it's a slow growing cancer, and medicine's motto is "more men will die *with* prostate cancer than *from* prostate cancer." The PSA test cannot distinguish between the tumor that will kill and the tumor that will not, yet a positive PSA test leads men to undergo surgery and radiation, which carry the risk of lifetime impotence and urine retention problems.

Ten years of screening data[68] reveal 1 man in 1,000 given the PSA test may avoid death, while 43 men will face serious harm due to treatment: 1 will develop a life threatening blood clot, 2 will have heart attacks and 30-40 will develop incontinence, erectile dysfunction or both. So "you go from being a guy who feels fine, and who is potentially one of the majority who would never have known they had this disease, to being a guy who wears adult diapers."[69]

Despite being "no better than a coin toss,"[70] emotion again trumps mathematics as pharmaceutical companies and the American Urological Association still recommend PSA screening,[71] ABC News reports "there is currently no overarching consensus on PSA testing" while the WSJ publishes an article entitled "Prostate Testing and the Death Panel."[72] Wrong! The PSA test harms patients through ensuing treatments, and doesn't improve the mortality rate of those patients diagnosed with prostate cancer.

The new recommendation is no man, should ever, take the test.[73]

The "Inside Job"

My brother is a conspiracy theorist and believes 9/11 was an "inside job." Conspiracy theorists have such passion for their causes, like Jenny McCarthy and her crusade to prove the MMR vaccine causes autism (which it doesn't[74]). It's too bad mammograms and PSA screening aren't sexy—like the CIA assassinating JFK or aliens landing at Roswell—because they are true "inside jobs."

Treating physicians should not have a say in screening criteria because they are not impartial: the more patients they treat, the more they benefit. Furthermore, being able to resect breast tissue or remove a prostate gland does not qualify a surgeon to crunch data to determine the inflection point, and age, that screening should begin.

Here's a policy idea (place tongue in check now): anyone who hasn't had appendicitis by age 18 should go straight to the OR and have their appendix removed. After all, a percentage of these patients will die from a burst appendix—so let's just take 'em all out. The mammogram and PSA debate is just as absurd.

And, if this can happen, what else do doctors get away with?

The "Next Step" Debacle

This relates to pain in two ways: 1) Tests we view of as benign—blood tests, x-rays, screenings—carry their risks unseen in the "next step," and 2) Even when there is evidence proving or disproving a test, unseen "other factors" sway medical decision making. If decisions at the macro level—nationwide—are affected when the data is transparent and convincing, what chance does a patient have at the micro-level—in an exam room—without access to the literature or knowledge of conflicts of interest? Data doesn't lie. But humans do. So get the data.

Nine major medical associations banded together (there's safety in numbers) to change the over-testing epidemic and published Choosing Wisely[75], a list of 45 over-performed tests no longer recommended. The few that relate to chronic pain I list below:

- Don't do imaging for low back pain within the first six weeks, unless red flags are present.
- Don't do imaging for uncomplicated headaches.
- A patient with functional abdominal pain syndrome should not have repeat CT scans unless there is a change in signs or symptoms.
- Don't perform PET, CT or bone scans for early prostate or breast cancer at low risk of metastasis
- Don't perform any routine cancer screening for dialysis patients with limited life expectancies without an indication.

Many recommendations were against doing imaging studies, because each x-ray and CT scan has a small but cumulative risk of life-time cancer. Other recommendations dealt with screening protocols not worthwhile if the patient is more likely to die from another cause that the diagnosis being screened for (mammogram and PSA screening were conspicuously not mentioned). The bravest recommendation was not to screen dialysis patients for *any* cancer, because their life expectancy is so short.

Doctors and patients don't plan ahead what to do when a test comes back positive, negative or indeterminate (neither positive nor negative). An example of lunging head-first into the "next step" dilemma are asymptomatic patients who pay cash for full-body CT scans to hunt for problems-not-yet-problems. A radiologist will always see some abnormality—a "shadow" or "density"—which then requires further "steps."

I fell into the next-step trap; burning pain in my groin, buttocks and hips led to an MRI scan. Six discs were bulging, so a discogram followed to "better visualize their internal architecture." A needle was inserted into each disc to inject contrast and the MRI was repeated, revealing the innards of the discs were abnormal (as we already knew). And that was that. They weren't planning on doing anything further if the test was positive, or negative. They were just doing the test. If I'd asked, "What will we do if this is positive?" and "What will we do if this is negative?" and they'd replied, "Nothing," and "Nothing," I wouldn't have allowed myself to be speared six times.

Dermatomes

Nerves carry pain and are two-way streets. A herniated disc in the neck (*cervical*) will cause pain down the arm, while a low back disc (*lumbar*) shoots pain down the leg. The road pain travels is called a *dermatome*, and a pain doctor will try to correlate the MRI scan with a dermatome map. Pain into the thumb (C6 dermatome) is a C5-6 disc, while pain to the middle finger (C7 dermatome) is the C6-7 disc. Pain down the leg, sciatica, doesn't map out tidily because the dermatomes of multiple discs overlap.

Dermatomal pain is a mini CT scan, pointing to the at-fault disc without the radiation. But with chronic pain the scan, complaint of pain and dermatome map often aren't in harmony; a protruding disc on MRI won't correlate with its expected dermatomal pain. The question then becomes: do you pursue the MRI pointing to Nerve A, or the pain that traces back to Nerve B? This question is answered with a drug called lidocaine.

Lidocaine

Lidocaine is a roadblock. Quarter strength solution is a flare on the highway, blocking sensation but allowing muscle movement. Full strength lidocaine is a spike strip across both roads—sensation and musculature—producing temporary numbness and muscular paralysis.

Lidocaine injections solve the dilemma of a MRI scan inculpating Nerve A, while the dermatomal pain maps out to Nerve B. Each nerve can be selectively blocked, and pain re-evaluated, to separate the red herring from the pain generator. In this way lidocaine injections are *diagnostic*; and if a steroid is added, *therapeutic*, by calming the inflamed nerve.

This lidocaine/steroid combo can temporize pain for weeks to months, to allow natural healing to occur. The evidence is strong that nerve pain from disc herniation will be the same after two years, irrespective of treatment[76]— surgery only increases the speed of recovery. Medium-term relief from the lidocaine/steroid injection prompts the longer-term treatment of nerve burning (*radiofrequency ablation*) or freezing (*cryotherapy*). This will destroy the nerve's sheath, stopping signal transmission, and provides long-term pain relief (6-12 months). It's not as invasive as it sounds, and if it gets you to the two year marker it's worth the risk. The "next steps" add up quickly: lidocaine injection; lidocaine/steroid injection; burning/freezing; surgery. Some pain clinics turn into factories: scan, inject, prescribe, repeat. Avoid these.

The Pain Menu

Knowing the next step—"What's on the menu?"—will make us more informed patients. Following is a sample of the common procedures performed in a pain clinic,[77] with the more invasive options in later chapters.

The three most common procedures—epidural, facet and SI joint injections—lack strong evidence; but this is different from evidence showing the procedures cause harm. Perhaps no investigator has taken the time, or money, to run a randomized controlled trial proving they work. An absence of evidence makes it difficult to give advice when confronted with all these procedures. Take two things into account: 1) the invasiveness of the procedure, and 2) what the "next step" will be if it's a success, failure or in-between.

The Epidural Injection

The spinal cord is suspended in fluid, allowing it to move to and fro with knocks and jars; similar to metal rebar providing horizontal give for a building to sway in the wind. This cavity is enclosed by a tough ligament, a wineskin, which lines the vertebrae of the spinal column. The bones are the structural cement holding the body erect, protecting the cord from rougher strikes and blows. Nerves cobweb off at each level, snaking through the aqueous medium, leathery ligament and shifting skeleton, carrying messages to the body's periphery.

The wineskin, the tough ligament enclosing the fluid and spinal cord, is called *dura*—and the space beyond the *epi-dura*, or *epidural space*. A laboring mother-to-be has a hollow needle slipped between the vertebral bones into this space, and a wire is threaded and left behind. Known colloquially as an "epidural," this beloved procedure allows opioid and local anesthetic to be pumped in, to seep around the dura and cross-cutting nerves, blocking pain transmission and the curse of child labor.

The chronic pain "epidural" is different. When a spinal disc bulges out (*herniates*), it irritates and inflames the nerves as they pass through the dura, causing pain to shoot along the nerve's path (*radiculopathy* and *sciatica*). An epidural is performed in this case with an anti-inflammatory drug; but no wire is left behind, and this one-time shot is guided by live x-ray (*fluoroscopy*) to better the doctor's aim. It's a shotgun blast, firing its pellets (steroid and lidocaine) in a large area above and below the herniated disc.

Patients have unwarranted fear of the epidural injection because of the proximity of a long needle close to the spine; but the needle is far from the spinal cord, and complications are rare: backache (7%), headache (5%) and fainting (2%). Less than 1% of the time a headache may last for a few days.[78] The evidence[79] for the chronic pain epidural is strong but the conditions distinct and specific—it provides pain relief for six weeks when a herniated disc causes symptoms of shooting pain (*radiculopathy*). The evidence[80] for pain lasting beyond six weeks, generalized back pain or chronic shooting pain, is weak or non-existent. The chronic pain epidural is an interim measure to allow time to pass and natural healing to occur.[81]

The Facet Joint Injection

Joints connect. Elbows and knees, fingers and wrists, ankles and toes. Two bones come together, the ends lined with smooth cartilage for frictionless motion. But each twist of the neck or bend at the waist put unsung joints to work—*facet joints*. Each spinal bone (vertebra) has four facet joints, two above and two below, to allow twisting and bending.

Trauma and time will degenerate joint cartilage, causing bone to rub on bone, and the diagnosis osteoarthritis. When this happens to the facet joints of the spinal column, the friction can inflame bypassing nerves leading to *facet-mediated pain*, or *facet syndrome*. This is diagnosed radiographically by a scan, or clinically by pain when pressing on the joint; under fluoroscopy a needle is inserted into the joint capsule to inject the lidocaine/steroid mixture, to both diagnose and treat the problem. If this provides relief, a repeat procedure can burn or freeze the nerves for longer relief.

If an epidural injection is a shotgun blast, the facet joint injection is a sniper shot. After the epidural, facet injections are the second most common procedure in chronic pain clinics[82], because back pain is the most common diagnosis, and imaging is so sensitive worn out facet joints are always seen. Back pain plus an abnormal scan anywhere near that level and the two are linked, and treatment begins. Never-mind the study[83] showing patients without back pain have as many abnormal MRI findings as those with back pain.

The evidence for the facet joint injection is inconclusive to poor. In a recent review[84] opinion was split—three concluded they were ineffective, and two concluded they were effective under tight circumstances (an inflamed facet joint on imaging).

My Next, Next-Step Mistake

Undiagnosed and hurting, I sought out the chairman of neurosurgery at my hospital. He noted my pain soured with position: bland lying flat, tart standing, bitter walking, acidic climbing and pungent lifting weight. This pointed to a mechanical problem—bone rubbing on bone—and the facet joints were soon indicted.

Over weeks he performed a series of injections up and down my back, left and right, alternating lidocaine and saline (salt water). The results: 100% pain relief when local anesthetic was injected into the bottom two facet joints; zero relief with lidocaine at any other level; and zero relief with saline injected into the bottom two joints (nixing any placebo effect). "We've found the pain generator," he said. I was elated.

Next was to still the inflammation with a steroid, but this logical step failed. This should have led to a re-thinking and re-evaluation; but I was in agony and didn't want re-diagnosing. Instead I gave the surgeon the tap he needed—all they need is a small push—and like a bowling ball at the top of Lombard St. he coasted the rest of the way, doing what he's trained to do—operate. He fused the bottom two levels of my spine to stop the presumed abnormal movement of the facet joints.

But these injections were a faulty GPS device, causing us to turn where no road existed. The injected lidocaine had spread sideways, numbing the nerves going to an adjacent joint—the sacroiliac (SI) joint—the true pain generator. When the steroid failed to ease the pain like the lidocaine did, this should have caused a re-evaluation (diagnosis, diagnosis, diagnosis!), not a brushing aside of a presumed red herring. I have myself to blame.

The Sacroiliac (SI) Joint Injection

The sacroiliac joint, or SI joint, is the biggest joint you've never heard of (unless you do yoga). It averages $17cm^2$ in most adults, and connects the tail bone (sacrum) to the hip bone (ilium), thus its name: sacro-iliac. It's deep inside your buttock and is a hip joint and a spine joint. In patients with low back pain, the SI joint is the cause 15-25% of the time.[85] And this is my monster.

It only moves a few millimeters, serving as a shock absorber for the low back, and shouldn't really be called a joint at all. It's injured with twisting movements (like my tennis), and diagnosing a SI injury is difficult because scans don't help. A SI injury, called sacroiliitis, is diagnosed only when someone first thinks of it, then tests the diagnosis with a lidocaine injection.

Nerves running to the low back, groin and pelvis pass by this SI joint, so walking with it askew (*subluxed*) irritates these nerves, causing low back, buttock or groin pain. Rarely does pain go below the knee with sacroiliitis. The treatment is the same lidocaine/steroid injection into the joint, followed by burning or freezing the nerves if the injection is successful. But this only treats the symptoms, and not the cause (the misaligned bones). I've never seen a physician assess the position of the SI joint by touch or try and relocate it to its original position manually. This is done by physical therapists, and only by the minority that practice manual manipulation (most emphasize strengthening). When my hip bone, askew for 5 years, was re-located to its original position, I was awarded with 70% pain relief. But it exposed a new problem, a hyper-mobile hip bone because the ligaments meant to hold it in place were torn. My hip continually dislocated when I'd go upstairs or carry any weight.

The four [86] RCTs evaluating x-ray guided steroid/lidocaine injections into the SI joint found the procedure provided intermediate (3-6 months) pain relief; but this evidence is far from definitive. A follow-up study of those who responded well were randomized to receive either a placebo or burning the surrounding nerves (*radiofrequency denervation*). Of this sub-set of the population, the treated group had 50% pain relief compared to 14% in the placebo group. This is moderate to strong evidence that in a carefully selected population, those with pain relief from a steroid/lidocaine injection, burning the nerve is a worthwhile endeavor (but this is still treating the symptoms, and not the underlying problem).

Make sure each "step" works before moving on.

Evidence Based Medicine

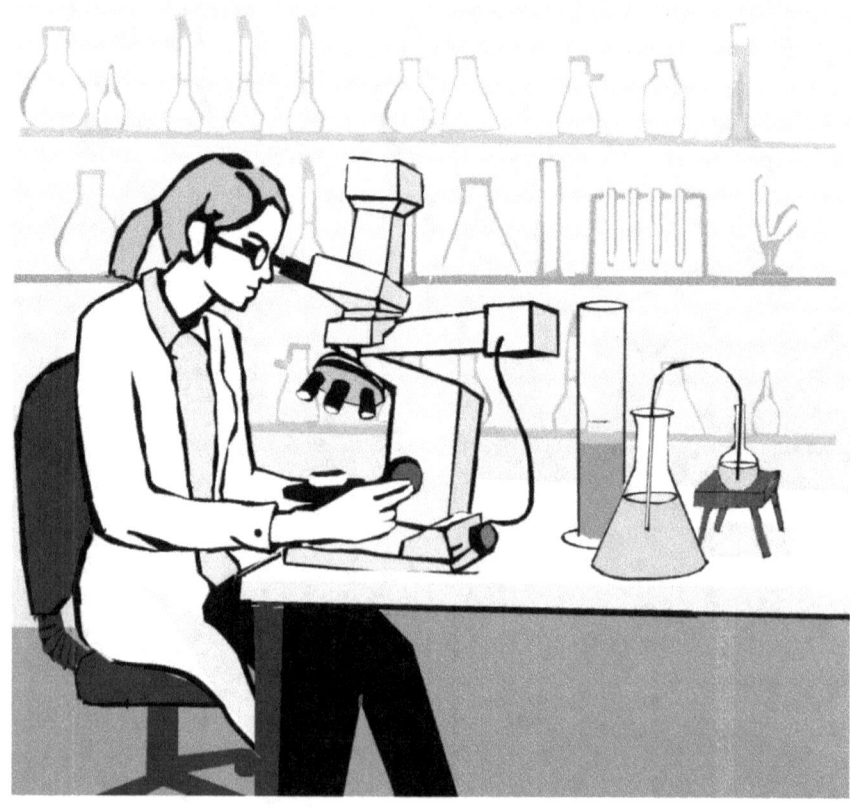

"Pleasure is the absence of pain."

—Epicurus

Apply for and obtain a home-loan and there's faith someone, somewhere, determined you're able to afford the monthly payments (or you'd be denied). Likewise in medicine, press for a treatment and get the okay, you have faith a physician reviewed your chart and concluded the procedure is warranted. In both situations the faith is misplaced and the religion wrong, because perverse incentives leave you at a disadvantage.

A bank sells the mortgage (and risk) to an investor, profits off the fees, and has no incentive to screen for risky borrowers. Likewise, a hospital and physician (the bank) have no skin in the game, assume little risk, while the patient assumes the risk of the procedure (mortgage payment). A doctor's reimbursement will jump from $300 for a clinic visit to $30,000 for a spine surgery (a powerful incentive). The stop-sign preventing this is evidence-based medicine.

Expert opinion medicine still runs the hospital, because trials challenging the standard of care are unethical (who wants to receive the placebo treatment for a brain tumor?), leaving a void of evidence. But evidence-based medicine is accelerating, and nipping at the expert's heels. Evidence often supports the expert—a simple aspirin decreases mortality of a heart attack—but other times evidence disproves an accepted treatment—a Nobel Prize was awarded for the lobotomy procedure. Treatments that appear medieval have been proven to work well: electroconvulsive shock therapy (for depression) and application of leeches (for venous stasis) are two examples.

A blocked heart artery used to require bypass surgery, which was replaced by angioplasty and stents, until the stents started clotting, leaving a confusing standard of care. The standard of care changes depending on what part of the vessel is blocked: an upstream blockage (called a widow-maker) requires bypass surgery, while a downstream blockage necessitates angioplasty and stent placement. A few centimeters one way or another separates a minimally invasive procedure through the groin, versus having the chest cavity opened and heart stopped in the operating room. For now.

Trials finish and standards change, muddying the waters and leading to "turf wars" as specialists compete for patients. A pain doctor will treat an uncomplicated herniated disc with steroid injections, a surgeon will treat it with disc removal and a physical therapist will treat it with stretching and strengthening. The three don't want to address the evidence:[87] doing nothing—a tincture of time—is the best initial treatment.

Laws of Evidence

Findings true today are disproven tomorrow. Here are rules that affect a study's validity:[88]

- The smaller the sample size, the less likely the findings are to be true.
- The smaller the effect on a field, the less likely the findings are to be true.
- The greater the number of tested hypothesis, the less likely they are to be true.
- The greater the flexibility of the study design, the less likely it is to be true.
- The greater the financial prejudice, the less likely it is to be true.
- The "hotter" a scientific field, the less likely the findings are to be true.

Sample size is power, because outliers have less impact with more participants. Studies evaluating multiple hypotheses have less validity than a follow-up study confirming a single finding of interest. Studies with unequivocal findings (death) are more likely to be true than subjective findings ("feeling better"). En vogue topics are less valid because of the rush to publish, as investigators compete, not collaborate: When James Watson was discovering DNA, he asked another department within his university to see their model to compare to his. "No" he was told.

Study Strength

The strongest single study is a randomized control trial (RCT henceforth): patients are randomly grouped to receive different treatments, with one group receiving no treatment (placebo), and all participants (patients, physicians and evaluators) "blinded" to the treatment each group is receiving. This removes selection bias (who gets into which group) and observer bias (expected results of a treatment). Randomization, blinding and the use of a placebo are required for a high quality RCT (level IB evidence).

Level	Type of Trial	Description	Question Answered	Example
IA	Systematic review, meta-analysis.	Combining multiple RCTs	Broad recommendations made on trends.	Raise screening mammogram age from 40 to 50.
IB	Randomized Control Trial (RCT)	Patients randomized into groups, 1 receives a placebo and all are blinded.	Does a treatment work? Does a treatment harm?	Ibuprofen works better than Tylenol for rheumatoid arthritis pain.
II	Cohort study	Follow an at-risk group and control group over time to determine the incidence of disease X.	What is the prognosis or incidence of disease X or treatment Y?	Compare smokers to non-smokers to determine the incidence of lung cancer.
III	Case-control study	Tracks subjects with a known exposure (smoking) against a group without the exposure to see their response.	How do demographics (sex, race, gender, etc.) affect treatment X in disease Y?	Nicotine patch works better for wealthier patients because they can afford to buy it.
IV	Case series	The symptoms of a series of patients with the same disease are presented in a paper.	Educational.	A review article.
V	Expert opinion	An opinion based on personal experience or anecdotal evidence.	"Doctor, what should I do?"	"In my opinion, spinal anesthesia is better than general anesthesia."

Science must be reproducible. Replicating a RCT ten times by ten different investigators in ten different countries adds validity to the results. A synthesis of multiple RCTs like this is called a systematic review, and if it combines the raw data, it's called a meta-analysis. The online Cochrane Library[89] stores systematic reviews for patient use. Systematic reviews and meta-analysis of multiple RCTs represent the strongest medical evidence (level IA).

Cohort studies (level II evidence) observe groups of patients over time to see influences linked to a disease. They look backwards (retrospective) by reviewing charts, or forwards (prospective) by following patients into the future. There is no treatment intervention or randomization, and a large sample is required to look for rare findings. Following populations of smokers and non-smokers to see the percent that develop heart disease is an example.

A case-control series (level III evidence) has a small to medium number of patients with the same disease receiving the same treatment, evaluated by how well the treatment works in relation to their demographics (age, race, sex, gender etc.). A study following smokers prescribed nicotine patches might observe patients with higher incomes are more successful at stopping smoking, because they could afford the patches. Case studies have smaller sample sizes, no randomization, and are weaker than cohort studies.

A case-series (level IV evidence) is not a formal study but a series of cases, usually by one physician from his practice. Expert opinion (level V) is the weakest and most prevalent evidence.

A review article is the best place to begin educating yourself, because it reviews the symptoms and treatments with less medical terminology because they are written for non-specialists. For each article ask: What type of study is it? How reputable is the journal? How recent and how similar are you to the patients evaluated?

Osteoarthritis

I will present the evidence-based treatment options for osteoarthritis (OA henceforth) to give you an idea of what's available. I divide, subdivide and subdivide again the data for OA until the best treatments are left. I follow the evidence as deep as it goes in the literature, to the corners only statisticians inhabit, to illustrate the depth that exists if you're inclined to dig thus.

Picking through a data pool with such thoroughness in a book for non-physicians may seem unsuitable. But when my pain was at its worst I followed the data to the nth degree (even contacting the authors of papers I read).

OA is not a new disease. The diagnosis and treatments for OA have been discussed since 1900: what could be left to learn? A lot. Between 2006 and 2009 there were 64 systematic reviews and 266 RCTs evaluating 35 different treatments.

OA is a "wear and tear" disease with the following risk factors: old age, being overweight, type of employment, family history and female gender. It affects larger joints and begins on one side (e.g. one knee), while rheumatoid arthritis (RA) affects smaller joints and is bilateral (e.g. both hands or feet). OA runs a multi-decade progression beginning with blood abnormalities released from injured joints,[90] followed by a painless stage with abnormal MRIs,[91] then a painful stage with abnormal x-rays. "Joint death"[92] and surgical replacement are the last phase. The disease is diagnosed by pain and a abnormal x-ray, years into its progression.

Following is the full armamentarium of treatments for OA from the most recent systematic review.[93]

Treatments for Osteoarthritis of Knee and/or Shoulder[94]

Evidence	Non-pharmacologic	Pharmacologic
IA	Self-management, Telephone, Education/Information, Strengthening, Aerobic and water-based exercises, Balneotherapy, Weight reduction , TENS unit, Laser, Ultrasound, Heat/ice, Acupuncture, Shoe insoles, Joint protecting braces, Electrotherapy/EMG, Surgical, Osteotomy	Tylenol (acetaminophen), NSAIDs, Celebrex (cox-2 inhibitor), Topical NSAIDs (Diclofenac), Topical capsaicin, Opioids, Injected steroid, Injected hyaluronan, Glucosamine sulfate, Chondroitin sulfate, Avocado soybean unsaponifiables , Rosehip SAM (S-Adenosyl methionine)
IB	Spa/sauna, Massage Surgical: Lavage/debridement, Patellar resurfacing	Glucosamine hydrochloride Diacerein
II	Radiotherapy	
III	Total Joint Replacement	

IB evidence (RCTs) includes randomization, blinding and the use of a placebo. Enough patients are included so outliers have no impact on final results. IA evidence, pools of joined RCTs, is stronger because it minimizes the impact a single outlier RCT will have. So let's snip off all but the IA treatments; this still leaves a lot of shrubbery. Comparing the effectiveness of weight reduction, acupuncture and NSAIDs is to compare apples, avocados and pears. But each fruit a common pit, and the core of the RCT is their use of the placebo.

RCTs compare their treatment effects to a placebo (treatment X works twice as well as placebo, and treatment Z works 5 times better than placebo). This common element, the placebo, allows us to compare apples to oranges, or steroid injections to opioids. A meta-analysis pools all treatments and their effects against a placebo, and calculates a single number, the Effect Size (ES henceforth). The ES is between 0 and 1, and higher numbers mean a treatment is more effective against a placebo than lower numbers. An ES of 0.2 is considered small, 0.5 moderate and 0.8 large. This creates a hierarchy within a hierarchy of Level IA evidence. OA causes three main symptoms—pain, loss of joint function and stiffness—and the ES of each treatment is listed for each symptom (e.g. opioids have an ES of 0.78 for pain, but 0.31 for improvement of joint function).

The following chart lists the ES scores in order for pain, joint function and stiffness.

ES$_{Pain}$	ES$_{Function}$	ES$_{Stiffness}$
Opioids 0.78	Heat/ice 1.0	Heat/ice 0.83
Heat/ice 0.69	Injected hyaluronan 0.61	
Injected hyaluronan 0.6		Injected hyaluronan 0.54
Injected steroid 0.58		
Glucosamine sulfate 0.58	Aerobic 0.46	Topical NSAIDs 0.49
Chondroitin sulfate 0.58	ASU 0.45	Acupuncture 0.41
Aerobic 0.52	Topical NSAIDs (Diclofenac) 0.36	Weight reduction 0.36
Topical NSAIDs 0.44	Acupuncture 0.35	Injected steroid 0.25
ASU 0.38	Electrotherapy/EMG 0.33	
Rosehip 0.37		Water-based exercise 0.17
Acupuncture 0.35	Strengthening 0.32	Tylenol (acetaminophen) 0.16
Strengthening 0.32	Opioids 0.31	
	SAM 0.31	Glucosamine sulfate 0.06
NSAIDs 0.29		
Diacerein 0.24	Water-based exercise 0.26	Lavage/debridement 0.05
SAM 0.22	Weight reduction 0.23	
Lavage/debridement 0.21	Injected steroid 0.2	Self-management 0.01
Weight reduction 0.2		
Electromagnetic Therapy 0.16	Diacerein 0.14	
Electrotherapy/EMG 0.16	Lavage/debridement 0.11	
Telephone 0.12	Tylenol (acetaminophen) 0.09	
Tylenol (acetaminophen) 0.21	Telephone 0.07	
Water-based exercise 0.19	Glucosamine sulfate 0.07	
Ultrasound 0.06		
Self-management 0.06	Self-management 0.06	
Education/Information 0.06	Education/information 0.06	
Glucosamine hydrochloride 0.02		

Abbreviations: ASU = Avocado soybean unsaponifiables; SAM =
S-Adenosyl methionine

If your predominant symptom is pain, you learn heat/ice and steroid
injections work better than ultrasound and weight reduction. If your
predominant symptom is stiffness, topical NSAID cream works better than
weight reduction. A low ES doesn't mean the treatment doesn't work,
because each has already been proven to work better than placebo in a RCT.
This is a re-ranking of everything that has already been proven to work.

When a rheumatologist recommends a joint injection, steroid and
hyaluronan are comparable for pain (ES 0.6 vs 0.58), but if the predominant
symptom is stiffness, hyaluronan (ES=0.54) works better than steroid (ES =
0.25). This is an example of how deeply ensconced data results in different
treatments. No physician is abreast of the literature of all the diseases he
treats. But you can read all the literature, because all you care about is one
disease, yours. Teasing apart the numbers may lead to different treatments.

Let's prune further. We've only allowed RCTs into our greenhouse, but
not all RCTs are equal. A JADED system scores RCTs from 1 to 5 based on
how well they randomize, blind and disclose patients withdrawn from the
trial. A JADED score of 5 is the strongest, so let's weed out RCTs with
scores between 1 and 4. This causes significant changes to some of the
results.

Treatment	ES_{Pain} (JADED=5)	ES_{Pain} All trials
Topical NSAIDs	0.42	0.44
NSAIDs	0.39	0.29
Glucosamine sulfate	0.29	0.58
Acupuncture	0.22	0.35
Injected Hyaluronan	0.22	0.6
ASU	0.22	0.38
Acetaminophen	0.1	0.14
Chondroitin sulfate	0.005	0.58
Lavage/debridement	0.11	0.21

Where to Begin

It's your physician's responsibility to be up-to-date on the literature for your diagnosis, so ask to see it, which will lead him to look it up and tailor your treatment accordingly. Living in the internet age, you also have access to the evidence. The two most prestigious journals, *Journal of American Medical Association* and the *New England Journal of Medicine*, allow anyone to search through their archives without fee or membership. Every diagnosis will have a review article every few years summarizing up-to-date evidence: put your diagnosis in the search bar followed by "review article" and see what pops up. The best articles are those written for non-specialists like family practice doctors, as the language will be easier to understand. Take the article to your primary care doctor or specialist for help in understanding the language. Remember the different strengths of the various types of studies, and take evidence with a grain of salt, as what's true today isn't true tomorrow (tell that to those who underwent lobotomies).

Aside from those two journals, I go to Google Scholar. This will search all journals for you, and allow you to view a summary (abstract) of each article. Most often this provides a sufficient answer to your questions. For half the articles you will be able to open a PDF or HTML copy of the entire article.

Association does not mean causation.

Five Common Diagnoses

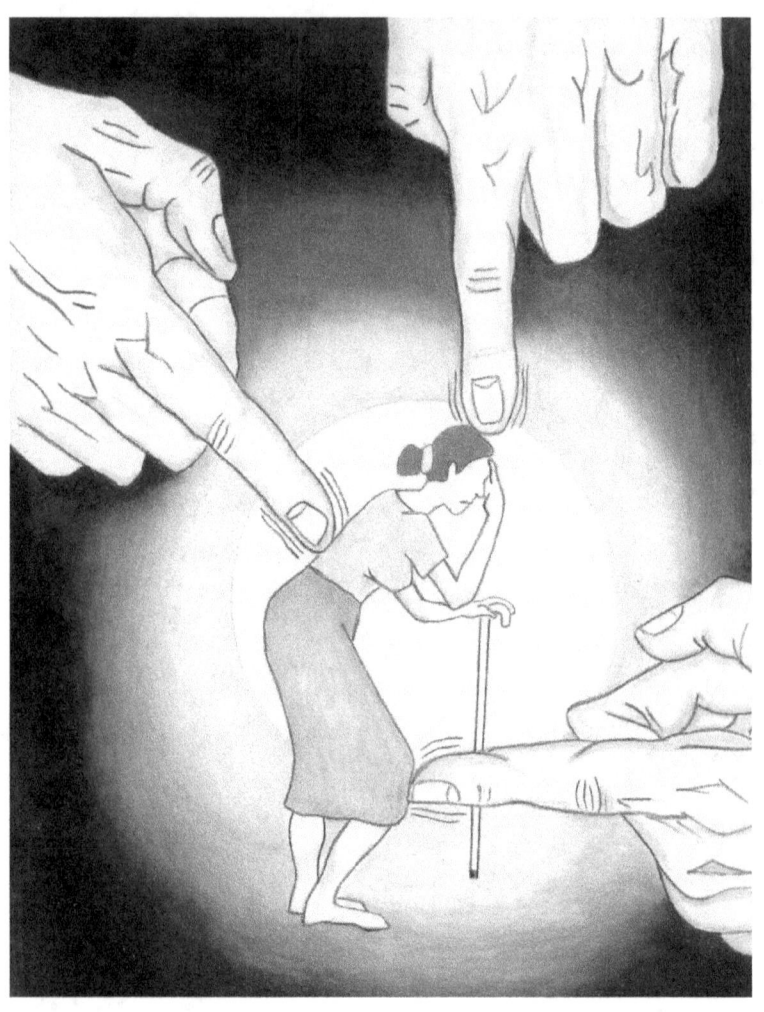

The five most common chronic pain diagnoses are fibromyalgia, joint pain, back pain, neuropathic pain and headaches. Each has subcategories that are treated differently, and the applicability of evidence from one diagnosis to a sister diagnosis is a conundrum in medicine, and a pebble in my shoe for this chapter. I will list the general treatments for the diagnosis where evidence is routinely extrapolated (e.g. neuropathic pain), and will pluck out one sub-diagnosis when evidence is not broadly applied (e.g. headache). Become an informed patient so you know evidence from sciatica applied to shingles is standard, but evidence from migraines extended to tension headaches is not appropriate.

Last chapter we gauged the depth medical literature goes: comparing the pain, flexibility and joint function of pooled RCTs for 35 treatments for OA. This chapter wades shallower. But depending on your affinity for data, the literature for each diagnosis plunges to the same depth. While deep, these waters are not still, as trials finish and evidence emerges at a furious rate.

Headaches

Headache, cephalalgia, is the quintessential invisible pain—skepticism is another symptom to treat for this diagnosis. Being up-to-date on the literature for headaches will convey credibility; subscribing to a headache journal is inexpensive, and will present the most recent treatments. 90% of initial headache consultations meet the criteria for migraine-type headaches;[95] but 42% of migraines are erroneously labeled as sinus headaches, and 32% as tension headaches.[96] Cluster headaches are the fourth sub-category. Treatment for each sub-category cannot be applied across the board, so I choose migraines to present here.

Initial treatment is ruling out a secondary cause (brain tumor, seizure, medication), and evaluating for any red flags[97] that warrant an MRI and spinal tap. Then the genealogy becomes complex. The migraine is a child of the parental category headache; the next generation, the grandchildren, divides migraines into episodic versus chronic and with or without a preceding aura (bright light).[98] The family tree widens as acute, chronic and preventive treatments are tested for each of these 4 grandchildren (creating the great-grandchildren, or sub-sub-sub-category). Then for each great-grandchild trials of individual medications are tested against placebo,[99] and the efficacy of proven drugs against each other.[100] If you have a headache that's a migraine, episodic, without an aura, and chronic, there may a paper written proving a specific medication works better for this particular offspring. Sequencing DNA is easier than tracking down this long lost child of a paper. A cobweb better describes such interconnectedness than a family tree.

Proven non-pharmacologic therapies include relaxation training, biofeedback, psychotherapy, magnesium, riboflavin, regular sleep, exercise and minimal intake of stimulants.[101] Evidence[102] supports early pharmacologic treatment of migraines[103] and combining treatments, because most migraineurs do not achieve relief with mono-therapy.[104] The pharmacologic treatments are in the chart below.

	Evidence Based Pharmacologic Management of Migraines
Acute, First Line	NSAIDs: Ibuprofen, Naproxen, Tolfenamic Acid Combination: Tylenol + Aspirin + Caffeine or Aspirin alone
Acute, Second Line	Migranal (dihydroergotamine), Amerge (naratriptan), Imitrex (sumatriptan), Maxalt (rizatriptan), Zomig (zolmitriptan) [Injection or nasal spray if nausea or vomiting.]
Preventive Therapies	Elavil (amitryptyline), Depakote (valproic acid), Inderal (propranolol), Blocadren (timolol)

Joint Pain

Joint pain has three principle diagnoses: osteoarthritis, rheumatoid arthritis and repetitive stress injury. Any diagnosis taken to its most extreme presentation is crippling (a friend of mine had ingrown toenails surgically removed). My brother suffers from repetitive stress injury; he injured his hip on a hike and was prescribed high dose NSAIDs for 2 weeks. He threw himself into his work, typing. After he stopped the NSAIDs, his hands were permanently crippled. The pain from typing, which should have alerted him to stop, was masked by the NSAIDs. He has to dictate even short emails. I presented OA last chapter, so will skip treatments for this diagnosis.

Fibromyalgia

Fibromyalgia is dismissed by many as a made-up diagnosis because its cause is unknown, its presentation varies and symptoms invisible. But within the last decade, gene mutations and brain abnormalities have been found in fibromyalgia patients not present in control patients,[105] legitimizing the disease among pain specialists. Unfortunately, this respect didn't spill over to the rest of the medical community, where stigma and skepticism persist.

Fibromyalgia is diagnosed by musculoskeletal pain at 11 of 18 specified points for 3 months.[106] Depression and sleep disturbance are strongly associated with fibromyalgia: 50% will have a major depressive disorder,[107] 75% nocturnal awakenings and 81% obstructive sleep apnea.[108] Other diagnoses loosely associated with fibromyalgia include: PTSD, joint stiffness, difficulty swallowing, bowel and bladder abnormalities, numbness, tingling, anxiety and mood disorders.

Fibromyalgia is common, affecting 1-2% of the population[109] with a 9:1 female to male ratio[110] (curiously 31% have restless leg syndrome).[111] I've known these patients through pain support groups, and I do believe in this diagnosis. To mis-quote Gertrude Stein—there's some there there that shouldn't be there.

Level of Evidence	Treatment Evidence for Adult Fibromyalgia Syndrome
I	Multidisciplinary treatment, psycho-therapy, aerobic exercise, Elavil (amitriptyline), Flexeril (cyclobenzaprine)
II	Lyrica (pregabalin), Ultram (tramadol), Cymbalta (duloxetine), Prozac (fluoxetine), Tropisetron, Balneo/spa therapy, biofeedback, hypnotherapy, massage therapy, homeopathy, meditation, vegetarian diet, whole-body heat therapy, written emotional disclosure
III	Opioids
IV	Trigger point injections, acupuncture, Tylenol (acetaminophen)
Refuted Treatments	Anxiolytics (xanax, valium etc.), Celexa (Citalopram), Corticosteroids, NSAIDs, neuroleptics, biofeedback or patient education as single intervention

Level I evidence:[112] a systematic review. Level II: at least 2 consistent RCTs. Level III: a trial without randomization. Level IV[113]: case studies.[114] Refuted treatments have been proven not to work.

Neuropathic Pain

Neuropathic pain, "nerve pain," is dysfunction of the central or peripheral nervous system, with symptoms of burning, shocking, tingling or numbness. It's precipitated by non-painful stimuli (*allodynia*) like a breeze or sheet brushing against the area, or exaggerated pain to something normally painful (*hyperalgesia*) like a pin prick.[115] Or it can just...be there.

Diabetes (diabetic peripheral neuropathy) and shingles (post-herpetic neuralgia, a reactivation of the herpes virus) are the two most common causes, followed by a long list of other causes: phantom limb pain, nerve entrapment, disc herniation, meningitis, epilepsy, hypothyroidism, multiple sclerosis, HIV, cancer pain, Parkinson's disease, complex regional pain syndrome, fibromyalgia, stroke and nerve trauma (particularly after surgery). Low back pain commonly is a mixed picture, with aching muscular pain and burning neuropathic pain.[116]

Medications for neuropathic pain work on different systems, so combining different classes of drugs is recommended.[117] A fast acting medication is started while a slower onset medication is titrated to a therapeutic dose,[118] and oral agents are combined with topical agents.

Medications do not cure neuropathic pain, and alleviate its symptoms poorly: less than 50% report satisfactory relief, and 30% have severe pain despite all medications.[119] Neuropathic pain is difficult to palliate, causing higher pain scores and requiring more medications than other chronic pain conditions.

Evidence from the two most common diagnosis, diabetics and shingles, is extrapolated to make recommendations for other sub-categories because of an absence of evidence. The strong,[120] moderate,[121] weak[122] and insufficient evidence [123] is listed below, along with treatments proven not to work (contraindicated).[124]

Evidence Strength	Treatment for Neuropathic Pain
Strong	Lyrica (pregabalin)
Moderate	**Antidepressants** Elavil (amitriptyline),Effexor (venlafaxine),Cymbalta (duloxetine) **Anti-convulsants or Anti-epileptics** Neurontin (gabapentin), Depakote (valproic acid) **Other** Opioids, Tramadol (Ultram), Capsaicin cream/patch, TENS unit, Dextromethorphan, Isosorbide dinitrate spray (nitroglycerin)
Weak	Lidocaine patches (Lidoderm), Psychotherapy, Acupuncture
Insufficient	Topamax (topiramate), desipramine, imipramine, Prozac (fluoxetine) Vitamins, alpha-lipoic acid, cannabinoids (marijuana), Biofeedback, Surgical interventions
Not Recommended	Trileptal (oxcarbazepine), Lamictal (lamotrigine), lacosamide, Clonidine, pentoxifylline, mexiletine, magnetic field treatment, laser treatment, reiki therapy

Back Pain

Back pain is the most common pain complaint worldwide, affecting eight out of ten people at some point in their lives. It has three sub-categories: non-specific muscular, nerve root pain (radicular) and serious pathology (tumor or infection).[125] Sinister causes can be ruled out by looking for these[126] red flags. The pain is then categorized as non-specific (vague in location) or radicular (shooting pain down the leg). Non-specific pain involves strained muscles and ligaments from heavy lifting, trauma or repetitive bending. Recent guidelines do not advocate a MRI scan for uncomplicated back pain.

A slipped, bulging or herniated disc causes radicular pain, shooting into a leg or arm. The disc encroaches on adjacent nerves, causing inflammation and pain along the nerve's path (called a *dermatome*). This most commonly involves the low back and the nerve in the leg, the sciatic nerve (*sciatica*).

Back pain is the most studied pain syndrome, but which treatment to employ when isn't straightforward. RCTs finish every year evaluating different diagnostic or treatment options. This diagnosis requires in-depth knowledge of recent literature, and makes the cobweb of evidence for OA and headaches look like a Monday crossword puzzle. With a multitude of studies to choose from, I'm only listing Level I systematic reviews (pools of RCTs); not teasing apart acute versus chronic, vague versus radicular and improvements in pain versus functionality (each has reams of evidence).

Treatments supported by evidence	Unproven Treatments commonly used
Back Schools[127]	• Epidural steroid injection[128]
NSAIDs[129]	• Facet joint injection[130]
Exercise[131, 132]	• Lumbar supports/braces[133]
Psychotherapy[134]	• Massage[135]
Muscle relaxants[136]	• Spine manipulation[137]
Acupuncture[138]	• EMG biofeedback[139]
Antidepressants[140]	• Traction[141]
Multidisciplinary treatment[142]	• TENS unit[143]

The general guidelines[144] for back pain are that patients should be given history and physical exams to categorize the pain as vague, radicular or sinister. MRI imaging should be performed for radicular or sinister symptoms, not vague pain. Patients need extensive education regarding back pain, especially in regards to self-care. First line medications for back pain are Tylenol or NSAIDs. Patients with chronic back pain should be referred to a multidisciplinary rehabilitation program that includes physical therapy, acupuncture, massage therapy and psychotherapy.

Learn the evidence for your diagnosis.

Down the Rabbit Hole

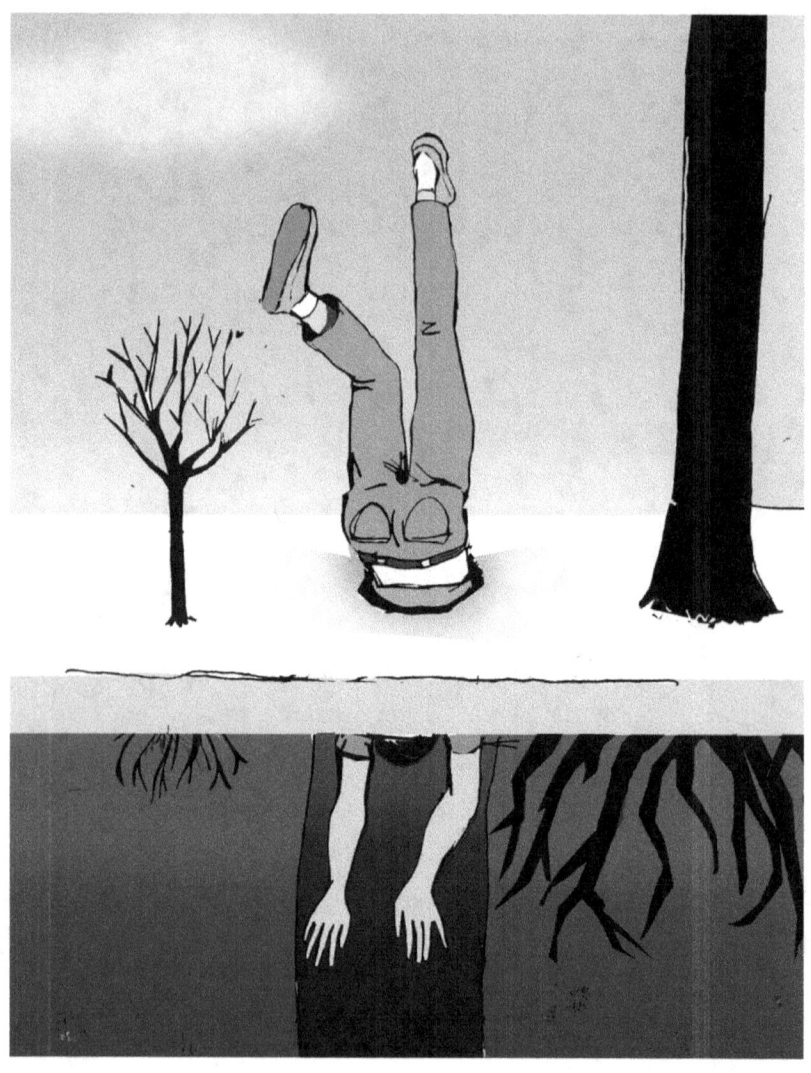

"I wonder if I've been changed in the night? Let me think. Was I the same when I got up this morning? I almost think I can remember feeling a little different. But if I'm not the same, the next question is, 'Who in the world am I?'"

—*Alice in Wonderland*

Alice fell down a rabbit hole into an altered reality of creatures with magical powers, ate cakes that caused her body to shrink and grow, cried, confessed an identity crisis to a caterpillar and attended a mad tea party. She was bombarded with riddles, and escaped to a croquet field with a domineering queen and a trial consisting of arguments over Rule 42.[145]

This is our new world.

We've been given drugs to change our bodies one way, then another, listened to dry lectures and had identity crises. A mad tea party tidily describes this new realm, with riddles (diagnoses) we can't understand, authoritative people (M.D.s) and arguments over our own Rule 42 (health insurance). We're down a rabbit hole; nothing is the same; it's *not* a wonderland. Alice's sister shakes her awake at the end of the story; but for us there will be no awakening, but the living of a nightmare.

Harnessing the Unconscious Mind

A nightmare is just an electrical impulse in the unconscious, sleeping mind. If Alice had decided she had the magic and was in charge, she could have willed away the fear, made herself Queen, and changed the nightmare into a dream. The world down the rabbit hole is altered, but equally important, alterable. It's malleable, and until the clay hardens we can shape and mold it.

Let's begin with the basics—the conscious mind. Information enters through the five senses, the data is processed, and we make decisions and act on this information. If we smell smoke, we decide to leave the building, willing our muscles to move.

One layer deeper the unconscious mind sees the same data, solves problems, store memories and influences our behavior, but without our direct control or awareness. The link between the conscious and unconscious minds is tenuous, but can be strengthened. The unconscious mind is a bridge between the conscious mind and the body's action system (the autonomic nervous system), which controls the heart's beat, blood pressure, breathing, food movement, pupil size and blood flow to different organs. We can't consciously make our stomach digest faster, or our heart beat slower; but the unconscious can.

Conscious mind ↔ Unconscious mind ↔ Autonomic Nervous System

Our mouth doesn't always water when we see a cupcake. The conscious mind first processes the image and alerts the unconscious mind, which decides whether to signal the autonomic nervous system. If we've already eaten lunch and aren't hungry, it won't activate the rest/digest system, and our mouths won't water. But if we are hungry, the unconscious does signal the autonomic nervous system, which prepares to digest the cupcake: saliva is produced, acid and bile squirt into the stomach, the intestines push food along to make space, the liver takes up fat from the blood and the pancreas secretes insulin. We don't consciously make our mouths water (or any of these other bodily functions); the decision is made by the unconscious mind.

Likewise, if we see a tiger, our unconscious makes a decision. If the tiger is caged and not a threat, the pathway isn't activated; but if the tiger is loose and poses a danger, it triggers the fight/flight response: increased heart rate, blood pressure, pupil size and shunting of blood from the intestines to the muscles.

The conscious mind filters what reaches the unconscious mind, which in turn is another filter to the autonomic nervous system and its opposing reactions (fight/flight, rest/digest).

						Autonomic
5 senses	↔	Conscious mind	↔	Unconscious mind	↔	Nervous System (fight/flight or rest/digest)

The arrows point both ways because messages go both ways: eat cupcake → stomach acid produced → stomach signals brain when the cupcake is digested → signal halts acid production. This back and forth creates feedback loops that maintain the body's balance (*homeostasis*). But the back and forth between the conscious and unconscious mind is under-appreciated, and under-utilized. With practice it can be harnessed to control pain transmission.

The Spotlight and the Floodlight

Freud divided the mind into thirds: id, ego and super-ego. Writer Daniel Kahneman[146] bisects it into System 1 and System 2. Medicine defines the conscious mind as working memory and the unconscious mind as procedural memory. But philosopher Alan Watts' analogy[147] is best—the conscious mind is a spotlight, the unconscious mind a floodlight.

As we shift attention throughout the day, the spotlight highlights each item we focus on. The floodlight (unconscious mind) is active without us being aware of it. As the spotlight highlights an item of interest, the floodlight illuminates the penumbra of our attention—the corner of our eye. Actions begin in the conscious mind, and are passed to the unconscious mind to free space for new conscious tasks. The conscious mind can only handle 7

(+/- 2)[148] items at once; more than this and it gets overloaded and performance decreases.

We can drive a car for miles while chatting with our passenger, accelerating, braking, and turning—all without consciously doing so. The routine of driving passes to the unconscious mind, while the conscious mind directs the conversation. When we encounter a non-routine event, the conscious mind re-takes control of the car: we hush conversations as we merge onto a freeway, pass an accident scene or approach a yellow traffic light. Have you ever noticed when you're looking for a street address you turn down the radio? We do this because the music takes up one of the 7 (+/- 2) precious slots of conscious attention, which is already multi-tasking turning, braking, accelerating and looking at street signs and house numbers.

The unconscious mind has enormous processing power and can handle more than 7 (or 9) tasks at once. Teach it fifteen tasks and it can perform them simultaneously; often better than the conscious mind, as is evident in sports. But it's an idiot-savant, yes like Rain Man, unable to teach itself or handle divergence from the anticipated path.

A woman on an airplane can knit, chat with her neighbor and order a drink from the stewardess without dropping a stitch. Her unconscious autonomously knits. But place her in a quiet room and ask her to knit while learning to play chess, and she'll be unable to make a scarf. Her conscious mind maxes out and disables the unconscious mind as it teaches it this new skill.

Athletes pass the tools of their trade to the unconscious mind; they enter a trance, consciousness recedes, and the unconscious mind plays the match. They don't consciously think which way to move or how to swing the racquet, the same way we can drive a familiar highway—turning, breaking, accelerating—without thinking about doing it. "Choking" during an important point happens when the trance is broken, and the conscious mind re-takes control. Performance moves from the better-trained procedural memory to the clunky working memory, and you become aware of every footstep and swing of the racquet. A procedural action becomes slow, deliberate and conscious.

I watched Andre Agassi destroying an opponent at the French Open, when a sudden cheer broke out as Bill Clinton entered the audience. Andre started missing every shot—his trance was broken—and lost horribly. Football teams call a time-out as an opposing player is about to kick a field goal (*icing the kicker*); their purpose is to move a proceduralized unconscious action to a conscious thinking movement. And it works! John McEnroe's temper tantrums win the trophy for this tactic, as his fake rage broke his opponents' concentration time and again.

The Floodlight

The unconscious mind processes information without command or awareness. I attended a party once, and as soon as the front door opened my mother said, "Something's burning in the oven." She wasn't consciously smelling, as we do roses, but her unconscious was whirring away, scanning and comparing all smells against a memory bank of known smells. The aberrant smell, burning, caused the unconscious mind to alert the conscious mind—the floodlight focused the spotlight. The same happens for sounds, textures, feelings, memories and thoughts.

The spotlight is a circle within the larger floodlight—one book within a whole library. You can speak to someone for hours at a dinner party, but later that night if your spouse asks what she was wearing, you can't remember. But your unconscious knows, along with the scent of her perfume, the taste of the food and texture of the couch.

Déjà vu is an explosion of recognition of the unconscious mind to something previously experienced. A signal of familiarity is sent from the unconscious to conscious mind, even though you can't consciously recall the experience (perhaps because you haven't directly experienced it). Perhaps ten years ago you dreamt of pushing a red wheelbarrow; then if you find yourself actually pushing a red wheelbarrow—boom, déjà vu. Seepage from the unconscious dream ten years ago connects the two events together.

Distractions and Filters

Hypnosis erects a bridge between the conscious and unconscious; and with a deep understanding of the interplay between the two minds, we can do the same while awake. Pain passes a signal over the unconscious bridge to activate the body's response system, the fight or flight component of the autonomic nervous system: an increase in blood pressure, heart rate, breathing rate and the symptoms fear, anxiety and irritability. Conscious pain creates an unconscious nightmare, leading to the body's signs and symptoms of pain. But we can use the conscious mind to influence the unconscious mind, and indirectly control the autonomic nervous system (heart rate, blood pressure, fear, anxiety etc.).

I do this with two techniques: distraction and filtering. When I experience pain I distract myself by working on a crossword puzzle, which saps processing power from the conscious mind (limited to 7 +/- 2 items). Go beyond this limit and you borrow processing power from the unconscious mind: As the woman learning to play chess can't simultaneously knit, similarly a busy conscious mind can't experience pain. The worse the pain the more complicated task required to bury it.

Meditation for me is putting together a piece of IKEA furniture. Some empty their minds; I pack mine full so no room exists for other thoughts—as I root around for pegs and screws the pain fades into the background.

Following written instructions is my chosen distraction technique for controlling pain; for you it may be meditation, yoga, exercise, acupuncture, massage or watching TV.

My second method of pain control—filtering—I use for anticipated pain more than averting present pain. Anticipation of hurt creates an authentic pain response. Focusing only on positive outcomes, done fiercely enough, decreases transmission of negative outcomes to the unconscious mind, blunting the pain-anxiety response. This approach seems shallow, but it works.

Two peculiarities of my mind stand out: (1) the conscious mind experiences pain but doesn't pass a signal to the unconscious (a good thing), and (2) being pain-free but having the unconscious rev the fight or flight response anyway (a bad thing). Through trial and error I've untangled these two conundrums, and refer to them as pain comfort and the pain-bot.

Pain Comfort

Feeling pain without a resultant pain response occurs in the absence of fear. Just as seeing a roaming tiger quickens your pulse, while a caged tiger doesn't, knowing the cause and duration of pain blunts the fight or flight response. The why and when provides comfort that the pain will eventually wander off, pain comfort.

I acquire this by inducing pain, then observing its severity, duration and quality with respect to that trigger. I repeat the process with the same trigger until I'm convinced I know the variation in the anxiety response. For example, if I walk uphill for thirty-minutes—a no-no for my injury—I will return home in $9/10$ pain with the fight or flight response: increased heart rate, fear, anxiety and chest pain. Knowing what caused the pain (the hill) and how long it will last (six to twelve hours) takes away its unpredictability, and fear.

It sounds sadomasochistic to repeatedly trigger pain, but discovering these bounds creates pain comfort. Explore your triggers and subtleties— how long pain lasts and how assuredly it disappears. You'll be surprised how calm you can be during a pain flair with this hard-won knowledge. What begins as distracting yourself away from pain with a complicated task advances to allowing pain to exist in close proximity, and being okay with its presence.

The Pain-Bot

The second quirk is the activation of the unconscious mind, and resulting pain response, while pain-free. Like post-traumatic stress disorder, but more complicated because of pain's deeper entanglement, it took years for me to decipher—I conclude it's due to a coding error.

Computer software is created by programming code. Occasionally a programmer errs and a bug in one line causes the whole program to crash. Or the bug can be maliciously inserted, like with computer viruses, and one hacker takes over an army of computers (creating a botnet, with each computer called a bot). A fight or flight response while pain-free is due to a coding error—a pain-bot.

A sight, smell, sound or thought can enter the back door of the mind (unconscious), initiate the body's pain response, without so much as rattling the knob of the front door (conscious). I experience anxiety-induced chest pain, while pain-free, by something that slips through a hole in my conscious radar, but gets trapped in the finer mesh of the unconscious mind. Pulling out the grating of the unconscious mind to find the ensnared item is a mind-bending task, because people, words, events, thoughts, images, smells, textures and feelings need to be dragged forth and judged as triggers or benign.

Twenty years ago a red wheelbarrow full of cement ran over my toe (not really), imprinting into my unconscious mind the connection of pain and red wheelbarrow (*synaptic strengthening*). Fifteen years later, if I see a red wheelbarrow my unconscious remembers what my conscious doesn't, and activates a pain-response.

Once I (really) accompanied a friend for a medical procedure and developed an anxiety attack. I was not in pain and had no procedures pending, but excused myself from the bedside as my chest tightened like a fist—PTSD without a known trigger. I was dumbfounded, felt like a poor friend, and waited in the lobby for the surgery to conclude.

It took weeks of rehashing that day to discover the spark that ignited that fire; and only by retracing my steps did I stumble upon the smell of the plastic IV tubing which yoked itself to the pain from my spine surgeries. My conscious mind knew a whiff of plastic didn't mean impending surgery, but the unconscious can't rationalize like this (the idiot savant). It's more like a computer you input with data and receive a response. But this computer had been infected with a virus, a pain-bot, associating plastic IV tubing with a scalpel cutting into my back. How to debug?

Trial and Error = Control

After unearthing how a smell set off a pain response, I rooted around my other senses to see if others would similarly betray me. The second discovery happened faster, as my two minds clued into each other. Driving by the hospital where I had surgery, viewing it for a split second, set off the next pain-free pain-response. Sweating progresses to palpitations, chest pain and a full-blown panic attack each time I viewed the building. Other triggers include seeing my stack of x-rays lying in the closet, the sound of velcro (used by my back brace), seeing someone walk with a cane or *any* discussion of back surgery.

From childhood we try and control our lives. Our tolerance to a lack of control is variable, but influences how we react to adversity.[149] For pain patients "feeling in control" is fundamental to coping, and wards off the additional diagnosis of CPS.[150] Patients who feel no control over pain develop learned helplessness, unable to perform even mundane tasks[151]

I now understand the interplay between the conscious, unconscious and autonomic nervous system; which gives me control to tweak the system. I've filled numerous notebooks describing my pain—even recording hourly heart and breathing rates after pain—and have a list of pain triggers and the responses they initiate. But I still encounter new triggers, and revert back to distractions and filtering as Band-Aids for these times. But then I explore the new triggers, and with experience, control them too. I no longer avoid pain triggers, but pull the trigger and live life to its fullest.

I'm in pain every day, but don't suffer from pain. It took a decade to incorporate pain's daily management into my routine—now as rote as throwing away old coffee grinds and taking out the trash. Your road won't be the same as mine, and you'll have to do the legwork yourself, but take the first few steps; prompt your pain, analyze it, and become comfortable with it—and see where it leads you. Harness the conscious mind to control the unconscious mind. But as you tinker with the unconscious, careful you don't bump into Alice, because you are indeed down a rabbit hole.

Deworlded: explore and control your new terrain.

The Opioid Escalator

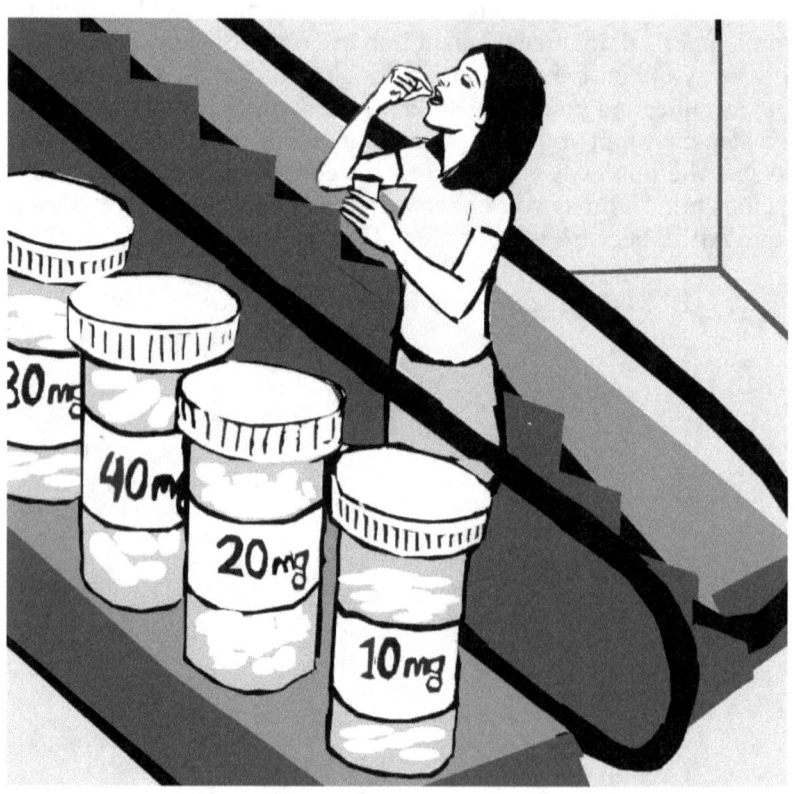

"Opium gives, and it takes away."

—*Confessions of an Opium Eater*, 1901

Every bump on the road caused searing pain into my groin. Scalding coffee spilling in my lap. "Shall I slow down?" my mother asked. A caravan of cars had accumulated behind us; I shook my head no. I lifted my body off the seat to create a buffer, but every wince was noticed. There we sat, two doctors in despair, with no treatment options remaining.

"Why not just take the pills and get high? Who cares?" she said.

I was puzzled to hear a mother say this to her child. Mothers across the world warn their children not to use drugs.

I was puzzled to hear a physician prescribe a treatment with such candor. No pretense of treating the pain—rather, "to get high." I had resisted opioids for so long, and now this.

I was puzzled.

Opioid History

Opium is a brown powder derived from the poppy.[152] Introduced to England from China, "opium dens" sprang up in major cities as tourist attractions, and "tincture of opium" became a common medication in the 1800s to treat coughing, diarrhea, pain among war veterans and the "travails and boredom" of Victorian women.[153]

Societal approval plummeted in the 1910s as immigrants abused drugs at a high rate, eased in the 1960s as Timothy Leary popularized "turn on, tune in, drop out," only to reverse again in the 1980s with the crack epidemic and Reagan's "War on Drugs."[154] Today's era, the 1990s to present day, is a nebulous time with disparate perceptions of opioids as life-savers and life-destroyers.

The chronic pain specialty emerged amid concern of the under-treatment of pain, leading to a patient's "right" to a pain-free hospitalization. Pain became the "5th vital sign," and broad expansion of legal opioid use followed.[155] Originally reserved for terminal cancer patients, doctors began prescribing opioids for *chronic non-malignant pain* (CNMP henceforth). As tolerance to Vicodin and Percocet developed, pharmaceutical companies met this new need with Oxycontin and Oxycodone. This "heroin in a pill" created a black market as "oxys" were diverted to the street, leading to an epidemic of abuse, pharmacy burglaries and overdoses. Sporadic prosecutions of physicians for overprescribing opened a debate: What is an appropriate opioid dose? There came an urgent need for medical evidence to "prove the practice" already underway nationwide.

What's the Point?

Why do patients with CNMP take opioids? To treat pain obviously; but pain relief shouldn't be the only consideration. If an opioid provides pain relief, but also incapacitating sleepiness, is this decreased quality of life worth it? Or if it causes an inability to concentrate, forcing a job change, is this decreased functionality worth it? Before beginning long-term opioids, consider their effect on functionality, quality of life and pain relief.

I once had a patient who was a competitive bridge player; his ranking plummeted while taking opioids, and for him this trade-off wasn't worth it. Chronic pain doctors don't treat the whole, focusing solely on pain relief. The time I worked in a chronic pain clinic as a resident, I never heard an individualized approach to the practical effects opioids have on a patient's job, family life or ability to drive a car (or drink alcohol). Mine is the perfect example: I was prescribed opioids as I sat in the clinic wearing green operating room scrubs, and a badge reading "Department of Anesthesiology." There was no mention of starting me on Oxycontin with a job where mistakes mean life or death. I didn't take them (then).

Opioid Dependence and Withdrawal

The body may develop a tolerance to opioids, but it will develop a physical dependence on opioids, and when the dose is lowered, withdrawal symptoms:[156] sleeplessness, GI disturbance, irritability, agitation, diarrhea, runny nose, goose flesh and a feeling of "impending doom." But don't confuse physical dependence and withdrawal with psychological dependence and addiction.

I was exposed to opioids after my first back surgery. My anesthesia colleagues kept me on high doses for five days, to not discredit our specialty if I complained of pain (as a bad haircut does a barber). After discharge I slept for 24 hours straight without taking any pills, and awoke covered in sweat, shivering and febrile. My mother took me to the ER and I was re-admitted. Infection was high on the list, and as I was pushed into an elevator one surgical resident said to another, "It's likely a take back to the OR for a wash-out." Being spoken of in the third person, while present, is a clear crossing of the line between doctor and patient.

The surgical chairman followed me closely, concerned. Leaving my room one day, I said in parting, "I feel I will die tonight." He froze, hand on the door knob. With those words I'd just diagnosed myself; I was in acute opioid withdrawal, and repeated verbatim the text-book symptom of feeling "impending doom." My body became accustomed to opioids while an inpatient, and when I was discharged and slept for 24 hours, the opioid level in my blood dropped and I went into withdrawal and right to the doors of the operating room. Luckily, I had an old cautious surgeon, giving credence to the saying, "There are old surgeons, and bold surgeons, but no old bold surgeons."

Tolerance and Hyperalgesia

The strongest argument against long term opioids for CNMP is they just stop working (56% of the time).[157] There are three theories why this happens: 1) tolerance, 2) disease progression and 3) hyperalgesia (a condition where opioids cause pain).

Tolerance is a desensitization of the body to the effects of opioids.[158] Patients quickly become tolerant to the euphoria of opioids; more slowly tolerant to the nausea, sedation, itching and respiratory depression; and lastly tolerant to the pain relieving effects of opioids[159] (tolerance to constipation never occurs, a constant companion). To treat tolerance the dose is increased,[160] followed by opioid rotation—changing dilaudid to methadone—hoping a different chemical structure will re-establish pain relief.[161] But failure of dose escalation and opioid rotation doesn't rule out tolerance, because some patients become so tolerant they never again attain pain relief.

Chronic opioid use makes any surgery challenging, because the standard treatment of post-op pain is opioids. Regional anesthesia—nerve blocks of the arms or legs, spinal and epidural anesthesia—is preferable for surgical patients tolerant to opioids.

The investigation of opioid tolerance then moves to disease progression—but what yard-stick measures the invisible? Pain has no blood pressure to check, or lab test to send off. If there are visible findings or an abnormal scan, these can be reassessed; but for most of us we just hurt, and then hurt more.

Hyperalgesia [162] is the third possibility, when opioids paradoxically cause pain instead of relieving it. If tolerance is a desensitization to opioids, hyperalgesia is a sensitization to opioids. This is diagnosed by withdrawing opioids to evaluate if pain improves (this is not a rare phenomenon).

Getting High

My mother spoke aloud what I had been thinking: I'm not happy with my reality, so why not alter my reality? I'd never been on a consistent dose of opioids, and my treatment options had dwindled; so with my mother's explicit approval I began opioids.

Rapture, ecstasy and bliss all describe how opioids felt (at first). It's a deep central nervous stimulation running the full length of the spine. I felt weightless, as I floated among clouds, with worldly troubles passing below. Opioid euphoria is Eden's paradise.

But it didn't treat the pain, it only made me indifferent to it. It was an incongruous joining of ecstasy and misery, like winning the lottery as your house burns to the ground. A calamity married to a wonder, but a net positive.

The Stigma

Chronic pain's stigma comes from this principal treatment—opioid painkillers. Mention chronic pain in conversation and you'll see visceral facial reactions, followed by disparaging remarks about "those patients." I experienced this firsthand when I filled methadone prescriptions; I had to drive great distances, and the pharmacists who did stock it gave me looks from over the counter, fearing I was the next drugstore cowboy.

I forgot a refill one week, and rushed to the pharmacy drenched in sweat. I queued in line, holding back the urge to vomit as the PA blared overhead: *Costco shoppers, we have a special on smoked salmon in aisle 24...*

I asked to speak to the pharmacist and told him I was in acute withdrawal and needed my methadone quickly. "I'm sure you do," he replied condescendingly.

Try our two-for-one exclusive deal on the economy pack of paper towels...

I lashed out. "Look at this incision, and this one. Do you think I'm taking these pills for fun?" I lifted my shirt and showed him the long scars on my back and abdomen (they went through the front to get to the back).

Free samples of smoked ham available in aisle 15...

Showing him surgical marks, and not track marks, made my point and he began to fill my prescription. But I couldn't let it rest. I blamed him for chronic pain's taint, and I focused my magnifying glass on this little ant.

"How would you treat a diabetic with a glucose level of 400 who needed insulin? Or a patient with heart disease needing beta-blockers? Why is acute opioid withdrawal any less dangerous?"

Enjoy a 10% discount on gasoline when you spend $100 or more on groceries today...

He was taken aback by the confrontation, and my knowledge, and the customers in-line perked up. I burned him to a crisp.

Chasing the Dragon

"You pay for every pill," one patient told me, and this is true—the initial rush is sublime, the come-down commensurately wretched. Each time you pop a pill your body becomes more tolerant, so you increase the dose, which helps, but doesn't quite get you there. So you escalate again, experience more tolerance, and a chase ensues. But you never "catch the dragon" (feel the euphoria of that first high).

Starting opioids is a weighty decision, because the time to physical dependence is brief. It clasped a ball and chain around my ankle; I obsessed over my pills, counting and recounting and matching each to a day on the calendar. Having extras gave me a sense of security, while one errant pill caused panic. They were my existence.

One morning, late for a flight, I forgot to take my methadone. I fumbled my way through check-in and security with a cane and back-brace as the sweating and shivering progressed. I made the flight, my arm hair standing erect, and as the plane taxied from the gate I reached for my backpack. I unzipped it to realize my pills were in the case I checked. The horror! The horror!

I was four hours behind schedule, and had a three hour flight ahead; nausea and stomach cramps came on as the captain warned of a "bumpy ride the whole way up." The turbulence coupled with the feeling of "impending doom" loosed Satan on this plane of hell. I stayed in the toilet 20 minutes at a time, filling the sink with bile from one end, and the toilet bowl with diarrhea from the other, as we rocked to and fro.

To this day I cannot fly.

The Evidence

Break a bone and you'll receive months of Vicodin, no questions asked. Carry any cancer diagnosis and you'll be slapped with a fentanyl patch; again, no questions asked. But procuring opioids for CNMP prompts skepticism and interrogation.

The evidence[163] establishes opioids work for short-term and cancer pain, which have the definite endpoints of cure and death. But the evidence that opioids work for CNMP isn't there, and doctors are leery initiating opioids for a diagnosis with no endpoint.

In order to prove a medication works, it must show causation—taking medication A causes effect B—which requires a randomized controlled trial (RCT). The RCTs[164] performed for opioids and CNMP have had three fatal flaws: 1) they followed patients for weeks, not the years chronic pain patients take opioids; 2) patients were on moderate doses, not the high doses we are ramped up to because of tolerance; and 3) the studies evaluated a mix and match of pain relief, functionality and quality of life using different criteria, making it impossible to combine the studies and see an overall trend (called a meta-analysis).

Nevertheless, follow-up of the patients with CNMP that *were* studied revealed 56% stopped taking opioids because "they stopped working."[165] They provided initial pain relief, but for the majority, not lasting relief. And evidence is abundant on the side-effects of opioids: infertility, decreased libido, decreased testosterone, physical dependence, tolerance, addiction, abuse, pain sensitivity (*hyperalgesia*), mental impairment and malfunction of the immune system.[166] There currently is no high quality evidence showing the efficacy of opioids for patients with CNMP.[167]

Pharmaceutical companies would fund a study to increase sales, and physicians would run such a study to stop criminal prosecutions; but the needed study is a RCT run for years, with few drop-outs or alternate treatments, and requires a proportion take a placebo. We are complex patients, jumping between doctors, procedures and medications in search of relief[168]—this study will never be undertaken.

The best evidence we have is an observational study[169] from Denmark (where a whopping 3% of the population take opioids).[170] It compares opioid users to non-users with the same *initial* pain scores, finding 90% of opioid users reported moderate to severe pain compared to 46% of non-opioid users (remember, they started with the same pain scores). The opioid users also reported lower levels of physical activity, employment, quality of life, self-rated health and utilized health care more than non-users. But this was *not* a RCT, and so doesn't prove opioids cause these effects, only that opioids are associated with these characteristics.[171]

Addiction

Addiction is not dependence.

If opioids are in the blood stream long enough the body becomes dependent on them. If the blood opioid concentration rises above this status quo level, you'll feel euphoria; if it drops below it, you'll feel withdrawal. But maintain the status quo level and you'll feel nothing. So driving, operating heavy machinery (as every pill bottle warns against) and even performing anesthesia is not problematic once a steady state is reached. Your feelings will change only when the dose is increased or decreased.

Addiction is the psychological drive to obtain a drug despite its negative impact on your life. Signs of addiction doctors look for are:[172]

- Obsession about future availability of opioids.
- Losing prescriptions.
- Misrepresenting how opioids are being used.
- Hoarding medications.
- Taking opioids despite deteriorating health.
- Running out of opioids early.
- Buying medications from the street.
- Exceeding self-imposed limits.
- Obtaining opioids from more than one provider.
- Spending excessive time and resources obtaining opioids.
- Lack of interest in other treatment modalities.
- Engaging in illegal behavior to obtain opioids.

Pain docs have patients sign contracts agreeing that if they show these signs, their opioid prescriptions will be discontinued. A minority of patients become psychologically addicted to opioids; but the risk is there, and addiction medicine[173] is a new specialty to treat the "opioid seeking behavior" of addicts. Methadone was the mainstay treatment for weaning people off opioids (and heroin), because it causes minimal euphoria and lasts for 24 hours, stopping withdrawal symptoms for that long. Suboxone is a new medication replacing methadone for this purpose. A history of any previous addiction—whether to gambling, sex, or alcohol—should disqualify patients from opioid use because they have an activated "reward circuitry system" in the brain, increasing their risk of cross addiction.[174]

A close friend from residency was caught using IV opioids intended for his patient. He was sent to rehab, after which he returned to work as an anesthesiologist (a mistake). He was soon found dead in his car with a needle in his arm, leaving behind a wife and one year old child.

Opioid addiction ruins lives, and entire families.

Walking Up a Down Escalator

If the pharmacy incident was a tug on my leg, the airplane episode was the entire ball and chain dropping off a bridge. It was also the beginning of the end of my opioid eating. Over months my body became accustomed to the dose, and the lighter-than-air feeling disappeared, leaving me feeling… normal—but in pain. If I missed a dose the shakes-sweat-nausea-doom-death cycle began. In summary, I had to take a pill every day that was difficult to obtain, gave me no pleasure, didn't treat my pain and whose only function was to prevent displeasure. Madness, I thought.

This is described as the "pain-opioid downhill spiral:"[175] the duration of pain relief becomes shorter, the dosage higher while functionality and quality of life deteriorate. I had trouble sleeping, concentrating, exercising and socializing, which I blamed on the pain and not the high dose of opioids. Each pill I popped gave me a positive psychological reinforcement, and my life becomes centered around doctor's appointments and renewing prescriptions—more opioid maintenance than pain management.[176]

I did not do what most pain patients do at this point; elevate the dose to recapture the wondrousness. I thought back to my training; of the bulging Ziploc bags of pills, with patients asking for more. No, I began the trek of walking down an up-escalator. But no matter how small I cut my methadone pill, I still began the shakes-sweats-nausea-doom-death cycle. I couldn't get off the pill that was made to get off the pill. How can anyone, ever, get off heroin? The horror stories of what addicts do to get their fix now made sense. I used a straight razor to shave the pills fractionally smaller, but there was no escaping Judgment Day.

It took six months to wean myself, and another six months to get over the mental obsession of little white pills.

Weighing Options

With the flick of a pen and tear of paper, you'll be given a prescription for opioids with a "let's-give-it-a-try" mentality. But you wouldn't give chemo "a try," would you? You'd get second and third opinions, do your own research, and come to a deliberate decision. Opioids are just as powerful, with competitive side effects and toxicity, so the decision is equally consequential. Take that first pill and you step onto an up-escalator, after which it won't be easy to change your mind about the "try." Weigh the risks and benefits of pain relief, functionality and quality of life for your specific life circumstances.

If physicians are to do no harm, prescribing long-term opioid therapy for patients with CNMP becomes difficult to justify. There are detrimental side effects and the best studies associate opioids with worse outcomes—overall there is an absence of evidence. Strong anecdotes live on both sides: lives ruined by opioids—my friend's overdose being the extreme example—and lives returned.[177] Currently more Americans overdose and die every day than those killed by gun homicides and car crashes.[178]

Perhaps our middle path—opioid acceptance and damnation—is the correct path. To err on the side of feeding the habit of a few addicts to avoid the tragedy of not treating a patient with life destroying pain. Two certainties exist: the decision to begin opioids should not be made lightly, and opioids should reside near the top rung of your "pain ladder," reached only after lower rungs have been climbed.

Opioids affect quality of life and functionality (and pain).

Alchemy

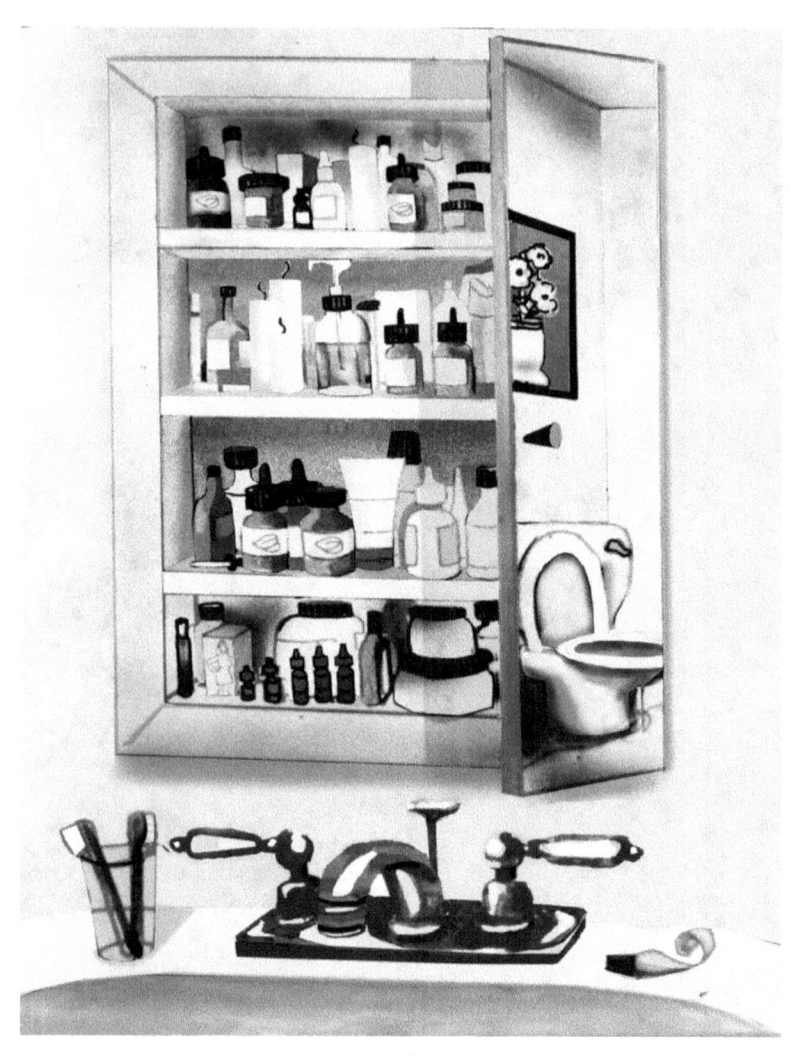

We all become alchemists, at some point. With so many half empty medicine bottles—not half full mind you, that would imply they worked—there's no reason to throw them away. What if we need them again? What if the right potion is mixing the correct number of blue tablets and red capsules with little white balls in them? Besides, there's no such thing as a real expiration date, is there? They just put that on there to make you buy new pills, thinking the old ones are duds. No, the left-overs stay as reminders of failure.

We keep adding to them, and they mount up, moving from the medicine cabinet to cardboard boxes. We combine like-types into bigger bottles, satisfyingly throwing away the empties. But before we do we scan the labels to see if refills remain—more pills to have in-hand. But if they weren't working as advertised, why refill them? As for advertisements, don't get me started. The endless side effects that accompany the man and woman holding hands, walking through a lush field, smiling knowingly (that he'll be erect when they get home). The listings are for the litigious types; but can't we sue for the not working part? That wasn't listed.

The Placebo Effect

Context matters.

If you see a doctor for pain and receive a pill, does it matter if he says, "This will surely help," versus, "This may help?" Or if you receive an intravenous infusion in the hospital, does it matter if the pain medicine is started and stopped without you knowing, versus with the doctor at the bedside informing you? In both situations the same treatment is being performed, but the context is different. For both, yes, it matters.[179, 180]

Is it a psychological phenomenon, or are there chemical changes in the brain producing a real physiologic response? What are the implications for the doctor-patient relationship, and how do we harness this phenomenon for the pain patient? Knowledge builds on knowledge, so let's start at the beginning.

The placebo effect was first tested with a sugar cube, with the clinician telling the patient it was a medication to help her disease. No matter what the complaint, the "medication" *did* help, and patients *did* feel better afterwards. The sugar cube was refined to a tablet, and soon research showed the shape of the tablet had an additional placebo effect: "Transparent capsules with colored beads work better than capsules with white beads, which work better than colored tablets, which work better than square tablets with the corners missing, which work better than round tablets."[181] Decades later the placebo effect is known to have nothing to do with a medication, because it also works for fake ("sham") procedures too.

A paper[182] aptly titled "Is there any point in being positive?" examined a doctor's differing attitude—a positive or negative approach—toward two groups of patients. The medical treatment for each group was the same, the only difference was the positive group was told their diagnosis was assuredly correct, and if a prescription was given the doctor said it will definitely help. The doctor told the negative group he was unsure of the diagnosis, and if a prescription was given he said it may or may not help. The medical treatment and makeup of the two groups were the same, only the doctor's words and approach differed. Two weeks later a significant improvement of the positive approach group versus the negative approach group proved a doctor's very words affect recovery.

This cemented the placebo effect as neither a medication nor a procedure, but the context of a treatment.[183] The placebo effect is "a positive context producing the reduction of a symptom." And context is a patient's entire milieu of existence: doctors, nurses, aids, pharmacists, pills, syringes, bedpans, neighboring patients, bedside manner—any visual, tactile, or auditory cue within a patient's surroundings.

The Nocebo Effect

The placebo effect has an evil twin[184] called the nocebo effect, where a "negative context creates the worsening of a symptom." If you think it, it happens. Women who think they are prone to cardiac disease are four times more likely to die as women in similar health who don't hold such views. Aspirin studied at centers where one warned of possible side effects and the other didn't resulted in the patients at the center with the warnings complaining of more side effects. Then there's the anecdotal evidence of surgeons refusing to operate on patients who think they are going to die, because, as one surgeon said, "Close to one hundred percent of people under those circumstances die." [185, 186]

The nocebo response is most applicable to medication side effects, because if you're told you may experience a side effect, you're more likely to.[187, 188] Attitude and mindset have a strong affect; the patient convinced no treatment will help, those expectations are met. All treatments fail.[189]

I was weeks deep into researching this topic and still had the gut feeling the placebo effects was a psychological response. I was wrong. Ph.D degrees have been awarded answering the question, how does it work? The placebo effect is caused by a release of our body's own stored opioids.[190] Opioids exist in a pill bottle in the medicine cabinet, but also within our nerve endings (*endogenous opioids*). A doctor at the bedside, and the knowledge of a drug being administered, causes a release of opioids activating the body's built-in pain relief system. The placebo effect is a real chemical change in the brain, causing true physiologic pain relief.

A parallel investigation studied the nocebo effect, also a change in brain chemistry. A protein (called *CCK*) is released that blocks the effect of the opioids released by the placebo response.[191] So the placebo/nocebo response is a balance between two chemicals, endogenous opioids and CCK, each affected by context and perception.[192]

The placebo effect has its greatest impact on pain, but there are other diseases it helps. Parkinson's patients lack a hormone in the brain called dopamine. Given a placebo and told the drug will help their tremors, they had a actual surge in dopamine in the brain verified by CT scans.[193, 194] The mind expected a release of dopamine, and so provided one.

Placebo Analgesia

It has been proven that open administration of a pain medication works better than the same medication given covertly. However, also affecting the pain response is the verbal statement that accompanies the administration; patients told they will receive pain relief required 30% less opioids than those not told this.

The studies I've cited are from the 1980s, but the placebo effect isn't a passing fad. A *60 Minutes* segment[195] in 2012 highlighted a Harvard psychologist whose research showed there was no difference between a placebo and an anti-depressant for patients with mild or moderate depression. He's not saying anti-depressants don't work, but that placebos worked equally well. Consider the impact: 17 million Americans take anti-depressants (including me), raking in $11 billion a year for the pharmaceutical companies. The psychiatrist on the show to refute the data agreed placebos were comparable to anti-depressants, "I wish our antidepressants were stronger. I hope we have better ones in the future." He argued anti-depressants worked 14% better than placebos for severe depression.

As I delve into in a later chapter, patients with pain from osteoarthritis of the knee did better if they only had incisions that were sewn right back up, instead of the actual knee operation.[196, 197] The expected healing from a placebo demonstrates the awesome power the mind has over the body, if only we can access it without trickery. But we can, and it's as simple as...better doctoring.

> [T]he doctors who prescribe the pills become part of the placebo effect ... 'A clinician who cares, who takes the time, who listens to you, who asks questions about your condition and pays attention to what you say, that's the kind of care that can help facilitate a placebo effect.'[198]

A rewarding relationship with a doctor improves health, while a confrontational relationship worsens it.[199] Find this doctor. Information needs to be given to patients before a procedure, but overwhelming them with every possible side effect will induce the occurrence of those effects.[200] Your interactions with the medical milieu affect your expectations and recovery from pain. I personally give my doctors permission to administer placebos to me, because I don't care how I feel better, just that I do feel better.

The main ingredient in the stew of pain treatment is the mind. Whatever you think is causing your pain, no matter how whacky, needs to be addressed: because unless the mind is set at ease, the change in brain chemistry caused by your expectations (placebo/nocebo) will lead any treatment to fail. I'm not saying demand an operation, but do demand an explanation why an operation wouldn't benefit you. In my case it meant one last CT scan to convince me my spine was fused. Before that, I wouldn't even listen to other proposals as to the cause of my pain. After my mind was set at ease, I was freed of an anchor—and the nocebo chemicals along with it—and able to journey on to new ideas.

Substance Abuse

Escape is why we are prone to substance abuse—to live in a world apart from the pain. And it does provide escape; but it insidiously takes over our lives. Like other components of CPS, addiction uncouples itself from pain and takes on a life of its own. During the occasional pain-free days, we'll still feel the need to quench our need for alcohol, opioids or whatever substance is chosen. It links itself to our personality, until we become both pain patients and addicts. We'll tell ourselves one is caused by the other, and when the pain is gone we'll stop the drinking, but this is foolhardy.

The lifetime rate of substance abuse among pain patients ranges from 23% to 41%, higher than the 16% prevalence of the general population.[201] I knew I had a problem during my fourth spine surgery. Keeping the surgery a secret from my family, I flew to Atlanta with a friend to help me recover. Before admitting myself to the hospital, I bought three quart size boxes of cheap chardonnay, which I entrusted to my friend to smuggle into the hospital for me during my post-op days. Being the good friend that he is, he pulled the plan off: my morphine pump was supplemented by white wine.

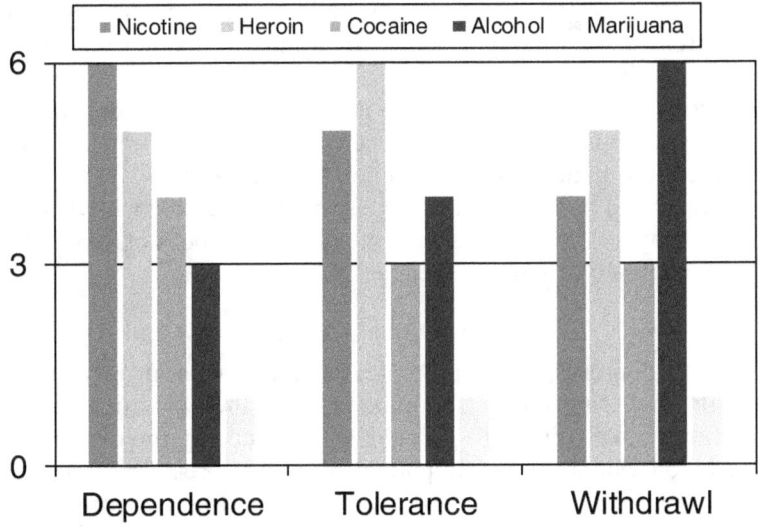

The bar graph above[202] shows the withdrawal, tolerance and dependence of the 5 most commonly abused drugs. These definitions are important to know:

- Dependence: How difficult it is for the user to quit. Includes physiological tolerance and withdrawal symptoms.
- Tolerance: A decrease of the effects of the drug due to continued use and adaptation.
- Withdrawal: Presence and severity of drug specific withdrawal symptoms.
- Addiction: A psychological drive to obtain the drug despite its negative impact on your life.

Two drugs of interest in this graph are marijuana and nicotine. Marijuana, currently illegal under federal law (yet now legal in many states) has the lowest level of dependence, tolerance and withdrawal symptoms. Conversely nicotine—oh so legal—is the most difficult drug to quit (even more so than heroin), and has high tolerance and withdrawal levels.

Walk the Strand in Venice Beach, California and you'll be steered into the "doctor's" office to get a prescription for medical marijuana. This country supports research into medical marijuana, and is prescribed for what it has been proven to treat: glaucoma, nausea from chemotherapy and wasting syndrome from AIDS. But it's currently "prescribed" for everything from acne to asthma. Evidence for these diagnosis is anecdotal—"it worked for my friend"—and not from RCTs. Try marijuana and see if it works for you it's the least problematic of all abused drugs. It made me paranoid and acutely aware of my pain, taking away my ability to distract myself; it shined a spotlight directly onto my pain.

The distinction between substance abuse and substance dependence is often confused. Abuse is a pattern of use causing harmful consequences: failure to meet obligations (work or school), legal troubles, reckless activity (driving drunk) and continuing to use despite these problems. Dependence includes two physiologic factors and five behaviors, but not all need to be present to be defined as being dependent.

Tricycyclic Anti-depressants

These anti-depressants (imipramine, desipramine, amitriptyline, clomipramine, nortriptyline etc.) are named after their chemical structure which includes three rings. They have been replaced by the newer SSRIs for pure depression, but chronic pain patients are often prescribed tricyclics because of their efficacy preventing migraines, treating fibromyalgia and neuropathic pain. They provide pain relief at lower doses than those used to treat depression,[203] but titration to an effective dose takes weeks and numerous side effects limits their use: dry mouth, memory impairment, constipation, drowsiness, confusion, dizziness, sexual dysfunction, nausea, vomiting, and irregular heart rhythms. It is also possible to commit suicide by overdosing on these medications. Tolerance to these side effects develop after continued use, and occur less frequently if patients are titrated to a dose slowly over weeks.

Anti-Convulsants

Anti-convulsants or anti-epileptics (Lyrica, Neurontin, Trileptal, Topamax, Tegretol) are medications usually prescribed to control seizures. Seizures are abnormal firing of the nervous system, and neuropathic pain is also due to abnormal firing of the nervous system, so they are cross-prescribed. They improve sleep, mood and quality of life[204] in patients with neuropathic pain. Side effects include weight gain, nausea, headaches, dizziness, sedation, lightheadedness and balance problems,[205] so these medications are prescribed to be taken at bedtime.

Topical Agents

Topical lidocaine patches deliver numbing medication through the skin, cause minimal side effects, and are used for localized pain.[206] Capsaicin cream/patch contains an extract from hot chili peppers,[207] and works by depleting the pain inducing chemicals (a process called *defunctionalization*). There are new topical agents that contain the active ingredients in NSAIDs. They are expensive, and I have never tried them.

Misc.

Ultram works via multiple mechanism and is less addictive than opioids.[208]

Medications

Every medication available in the pharmacy we already have available in our bodies. We have to, because in order for a medication to work, our cells must have receptors that match that drug. Anti-depressants affect the serotonin, dopamine and epinephrine receptors. Benzodiazepines activate the GABA receptor.

Surgery #1

Back pain is my monster, so its emphasized in this chapter. I had disc bulges, degenerative changes and curious shadows on my MRI, and didn't fit into the back pain algorithm because I had burning pain in my groin and butt without low back pain or radicular pain shooting below the knee. The assumption was it was spine related, and so I had an eight month trial of NSAIDs, opioids, steroid facet injections, epidural injections and even a 6 level discogram. I didn't try physical therapy or psychotherapy—the two multidisciplinary elements that ended up helping the most. Not fitting neatly into the back pain category, I jumped onto the neuropathic pain pathway: This led to different medication trials—Neurontin, Lyrica, anti-seizure drugs, anti-depressants, lidocaine patches, capsaicin cream and a long acting opioid, methadone. Nothing helped, and I was lost between categories, not knowing which specialist to see.

I jumped back to the back pain pathway (does this sound familiar?) and repeated the injections—and lidocaine injected into the lower back joints provided pain relief. I latched onto this wisp of hope, had the injections repeated while blinded to which joints were being injected with lidocaine versus saline. And again, injection of lidocaine into the lower two facet joints provided pain relief.

I had waited two years, well beyond the requisite time to allow a natural cure from a herniated disc, and still couldn't walk, lift a gallon of milk, or get up from the couch as every movement caused my constant 8/10 pain to jump to 10/10. I was presented at multiple "grand rounds" and discussed between disciplines, finally turning to the chairman of neurosurgery at the best institution in the nation, begging for "a try." I proceeded with a lumbar fusion under the hypothesis that abnormal movement of the bottom two facet joints was causing my pain. Complications ensued—urinary retention, pneumonia, opioid withdrawal—and it ultimately took a second surgery to definitively fuse those bottom two joins. I'd been on disability for 3-4 years by this point, and depression and anxiety became overwhelming, leading to my referral to a multidisciplinary pain center, and where I continue my story in "Team Treatment."

Two spinal fusions over three years put me into a constant post-op recovery state. The golden rule after spinal fusion is "no bending, twisting, or lifting," as you don't want to put stress on the newly unionized bones: Over three months, small bony bridges form, permanently cementing the spine together. You'll need to get creative to follow these rules. How do you pick up the toilet seat? How do you get your morning paper? You'll find you can't empty the dishwasher or put your socks on in the morning.

First thing you'll need is a "pickup stick"—sold on Amazon.com for $25. It's an extension of your arm with a mechanical claw at the end. I used it for everything: adjusting the hot and cold water while in the bath, picking up laundry, emptying the bottom rack of the dishwasher, getting the newspaper from the curb and yes, even raising the toilet seat. The shoelace and sock issue took longer to solve: I switched to slip on shoes, avoiding shoelaces altogether, and eventually discovered another device called a sock-donner—a tubular device with straps allowing you to pull your socks on without bending at the waist.

Nifty devices aside, you will have to give up certain activities for a long period of time after surgery. Lifting heavy objects is the most significant. There is no innovative solution except to pull a basket with wheels on it. Grocery shopping will be difficult: How do you get a twelve-pack of soda into the car? I turned to the Internet and Safeway's online delivery. For $8 they will deliver your groceries to your front door. And for a tip, they will even put the heavy items into the fridge for you.

I recommend getting a handicapped parking placard before surgery so it's ready for your six weeks of recovery. There is reciprocity from state to state, and it helps in two ways: you gain access to the blue reserved spaces, and no longer have to pay parking meters. A caregiver is the last must-have during this period. Recovering from back surgery is one big fiddle-faddle as you encounter taken-for-granted activities that now befuddle you.

Mix your match, and remember: Context matters.

Team Treatment

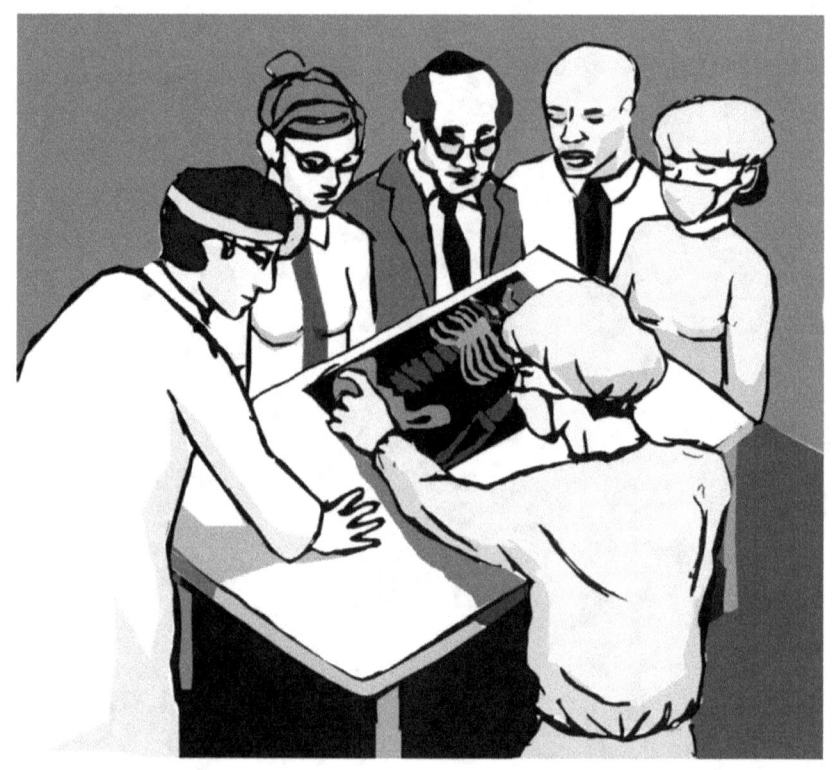

"The cure of the part should not be attempted without treatment of the whole. No attempt should be made to cure the body without the soul and, if the head and body are to be healthy, you must begin by curing the mind. … for this is the great error of our day in the treatment of the human body, the physicians first separate the soul from the body."

—Plato, fifth century BC

This chapter was first titled Biopsychosocial, but renamed after my brother, the illustrator, complained he couldn't depict a word he couldn't understand—such is the difficulty I have explaining the best treatment for chronic pain. The biopsychosocial treatment model veers from the "uniformity myth"—the hammer and nail approach of prescribing treatment X for diagnosis Y—and instead focuses on tailoring the treatment to the patient. Emphasis is placed on collaboration, treatment customization, flexibility, acceptance, coping and resourcefulness (over denial, cure and helplessness).[209]

Pain is best treated with a team approach for the pathologic (bio), psychologic (psycho) and social components (bio-psycho-social) that require individual attention. Since multiple diagnoses stem from Chronic Pain Syndrome—anxiety, depression, substance abuse, catastrophizing, social isolation, personality disorders, sleep disturbance and opioid dependence—this model just makes sense.

Anxiety and depression are the top two co-diagnoses, so referral to both a psychologist and psychiatrist is proper. Pain restricts physical activities causing muscular deconditioning, social isolation and depression. A physical therapist can reverse these. Psychologist, pain doctor and physical therapist are the three legs of a stool that make up the core team for the chronic pain patient.

Then, depending on the character of pain, seeing a specialist of that discipline is appropriate: Pain is transmitted through nerves, so evaluation by a neurologist is fitting. We become disabled, tussle with insurance companies and the needs of family life—here a social worker lends aid. Passing one day with chronic pain is an obstacle course, but an occupational therapist's knowledge-set lowers the bar and shortens the race. The pelvic pain patient should see a gynecologist; the cancer patient a hospice physician; the joint pain patient a rheumatologist; the abdominal pain patient a gastroenterologist; and the foot pain patient a podiatrist.

At the core of the Biopsychosocial Model[210] is the primary pathology precipitating the pain, and all that it entails: doctor appointments, medications, surgeries and procedures. All of this affects our psychological well-being, the larger circle within which the components of the Chronic Pain Syndrome reside. And the pathological pain and psychological stressors live within the larger social milieu of work, family, relationships and finances.

Multidisciplinary

I knew multidisciplinary chronic pain programs existed because the hospital I trained at had one, but I didn't know private programs also existed, until I was referred to one. The intake evaluation lasted a full day. I was evaluated by a physical therapist, psychologist, occupational therapist and a Physical Medicine and Rehabilitation (PMNR) doctor. My expectations were low, as I arrogantly thought: I know more about pain management than these people.

I met first with the psychologist, who had me fill out a lengthy questionnaire. He spent an hour interviewing me, with each question slanted towards pain: What were my coping mechanisms for pain? I don't have any. How does my anxiety and depression correlate with my pain level? I've never thought of that. How has pain affected my life? My answer: tears. He asked questions to which I didn't know answers, but felt I should. This peculiar therapy session foreshadowed the bizarre day that was to come.

Next I saw an occupational therapist, who also impressed me by knowing the motions I struggled with—bending, twisting and lifting. Her questions exposed my lack of knowledge, and her expertise. Why haven't I exchanged my soft couch for a firm one? Why do I still use the bottom rack of the dishwasher? Have I considered changing my side-by-side refrigerator to a top-bottom model? Do I have a firm seat insert for public places like movie theaters?

The PMNR doc then took his turn, going over my history in detail. Every misdiagnosis and ineffective surgery, procedure and medication that in my mind represented medical debacles, in his mind were puzzle pieces that fit in place. He didn't shake his head in disapproval, but nodded in understanding. He'd seen it all before. I presented my X-rays, which he waved off (Huh? Those are the first thing doctors ask for). He took an unconventional history. What extracurricular activities did I do? Who were my friends? What exercise did I do? Did I drink? And his last question was the furthest afield: Did I accept my pain? No, I didn't. That's why I'm here, for you to cure this fucking problem. He smiled and nodded, leaving me outside an inside joke.

Then came Janelle, the physical therapist. I shook my head in disapproval because she looked to be 25, but was surprised as she firmly took control. She knew my history and dove into the physical exam, the most intimate I've ever experienced. She palpated the contours of my hip bones with her fingers, not slowing down as she got close to my groin, but proceeding along every bony protuberance. I was astonished, but did as she asked. She confidently declared, "You have a sacroiliac joint problem." Yeah right, you've figured out in 5 minutes what the brightest minds at the country's best hospital couldn't over 6 years. Reading my mind, and to prove her point, she lay me flat on my back and pointed to my feet, "See, one leg is longer than the other." And she was right; the heel of one foot was half a foot below the heel of the other. She then sat me upright, causing my legs to equalize in length.

My head spun as I tried to take this in, but there was no slowing her down. She wrapped a towel around one ankle and told me to relax. I asked what she was doing, and she said she couldn't tell me because it wouldn't work if I knew. What kind of medicine was this? Minutes passed with us looking at each other, Janelle standing at the foot of the bed with a towel wrapped around an ankle. I soon turned my head to look around the room, at which point she yanked downward as hard as possible. Then her hands went back to my groin, feeling around. Shaking her head, she said, "It didn't work," walking away without explanation.

I was exhausted after these back-to-back appointments. I sat in a room as the four evaluators gave their opinion. I was a "classic chronic pain patient" they agreed, a typical case. The psychologist said I was at the extreme end in regards to anxiety and depression, neither of which had been addressed in the slightest, and I had other aspects of the Chronic Pain Syndrome (social withdrawal and alcohol abuse).

The PMNR doctor thought I was a perfect candidate for the program, but had a long way to go. "Health care workers are the most difficult patients because they so focus on cure, not coping. He's a long way from acceptance," he said, referring to me in the third person, implicitly implying I disagreed with him. I did.

This one-story private pain program seemed to relish the poor care I had received up until now, smirking every time my hospital's top notch-name was mentioned. The occupational therapist listed the ergonomic changes she recommended; finally, something I agreed with.

And Janelle spoke last—who had touched me so intimately, then roughly—and the room went quiet, as if she deserved special deference. She said I had classic SI joint pathology with an abnormally rotated pelvic bone, askew for years, that she couldn't pull down to its original position. She said she had a lot of work to do on me.

Then an administrator told me my insurance had agreed to cover the cost for 2 weeks, beginning Monday. I agreed, and was soon driving home, trying to take in the singular experience I had just witnessed.

Janelle

For two weeks I attended the pain center, every window curtained with forest greenery. The psychologist emphasized a long-term relationship with one therapist experienced with chronic pain, providing a list of providers to interview. The occupational therapist taught me how to make my environment "back friendly": install an elevated front load washer and dryer, a top-bottom refrigerator, a dishwasher with two separate pull-out drawers, a sit-stand desk that can be raised and a back-up camera in my car to prevent twisting when reversing. I attended group classes on coping and distraction techniques. But Janelle changed my life.

She taught me about the SI joint, and I was an eager student. I had dissected a cadaver in medical school, but my knowledge of this joint was lacking. It moves only a few millimeters and is a shock absorber, protecting the back by absorbing the jars of walking.

She likened the joint to two bananas lying side by side, one representing the sacrum (tail bone) and the other the hip bone. Most joints move in a two-dimensional plane, forward and backward, like the knee and elbow. But the SI joint moves in a three-dimensional plane, through six directions: up and down (upslip or downslip), rotated forward or backwards (anterior or posterior rotation) and side to side (called flair).

Ligaments and muscles cross the joint and hold the bones in place. The classic injury is stepping off an unseen curb; one leg plunges lower than the other, pulling the hip bone and rotating it (so the bananas are no longer side by side, but askew). When lying flat, a rotated hip bone will cause one leg to be longer than the other. A physical therapist can rotate the hip bone back to its original position, re-positioning the bananas side by side (but the majority of PTs don't perform manual manipulations).

Janelle taught me to assess the position of my hip bone, demonstrating my right hip bone had an upslip, anterior rotation and flair. It was off in all three dimensions, and had been so for a long time (with time, make that four dimensions). She again yanked my leg down to try and rotate my hip back, but couldn't budge it. But I left elated. Was this finally the cause of my pain? I spent days reading every article written about the SI joint, and told her of my plan to pull my hip down to its proper position—an inversion table. You strap your feet into this machine and it flips you upside down, so you hang by your ankles. She said to try it; so I bought a used inversion table off the internet. I was wary of yet another diagnosis, but the leg length difference was remarkable, and unarguably abnormal.

I strapped my feet into the inversion table and tilted myself upside down, a few degrees at a time. Soon I was hanging upside down as the blood rushed to my head. It stretched my back nicely, but there was no movement of my hip. I returned to Craigslist and bought some barbells. I then hung upside down again and held the weights against my chest, and felt a sudden give. I got off, lay flat on the ground, and checked my leg length. It was improved. I got back into the machine, grabbed the barbells, and this time hung by my one bad leg, which produced even more movement in my pelvis. I swung back, and before I could even unstrap myself, my constant seven-year pain had dropped from $8/_{10}$ to $4/_{10}$. I lay flay—my legs were the same length!

The next morning I told Janelle, and she winced as I told her I hung upside down, by one leg, holding barbells. Yet her concern dissolved as she began her routine of palpation, declaring my upslip corrected. I still had some flair and rotation, and we began manual manipulations to correct these. I learned how to check the position of my pelvis, and self-correct for a rotation and flair.

But no sooner was one problem solved when another reared its head; every time I went up a step, or walked carrying even a few ounces, I felt my hip "go out," and the $^8/_{10}$ pain returned. My hip kept dislocating and rotating—a partial dislocation is called subluxation—and I'd have to manually relocate it. This continued month after month as I worked on strengthening the muscles of the hip and pelvis. Yet no matter how hard I worked, I couldn't stop subluxing from the slightest movement, which caused my pain to jump from 4 to 8. I had made an important step in being diagnosed correctly; unfortunately, actual steps caused me to regress.

Janelle taught me to "step up with the good and down with the bad," which helped, but avoided the problem of my hip bone not holding itself in position. I began wearing a SI belt: you wear this a few inches below your waist line to hold the hips in position. I bought every SI belt sold, but they were all too wide, because it was intended to fit into the small notch underneath the front of the pelvis. I therefore made my own SI belts, hiring a leather-smith to craft one with sheepskin on the interior for padding. I'd cinch this thin belt as tight as possible, and got through the day with only 5-8 dislocations of my hip.

I began using a cane to take weight off my bad hip, which Janelle saw as moving in the wrong direction. But she had moved me far in the correct direction, and I didn't see it this way. I couldn't decrease the subluxations to less than five a day, each time requiring me to lay on my back and rotate the hip back to its original position. Janelle said the ligaments were stretched and would tighten over time; but after a year I gave up on this idea, convinced the ligaments were torn. It's a close call, but the prior constant $^8/_{10}$ pain was better than the continual dislocations of my hip. My pain improved as my disability level worsened. Another calamity married to a wonder, but this time a net negative. Janelle discharged me after a year, still wearing the SI belt and walking with two canes. Yet no matter how much strengthening I did, I couldn't get the hip to stay in place. So I turned again to the knife.

Fear and Avoidance

Pain = Harm. This is a logical assumption to make, as pain's purpose is to steer us away from harm, and acute pain does correlate with tissue injury (the longer you touch something hot, the worse the burn will be). But chronic pain persists beyond its useful protective period, and the correlation between pain and harm loses its association. The chronic pain patient needs to deprogram the mindset, albeit a logical one, of pain = injury, and reprogram: pain ≠ harm.[211]

The chronic pain patient refuses to travel for fear of reinjury; she is restricted not by pain, but by fear of pain. Avoiding traveling, or doing things, does not improve her everyday pain, and the avoidant behavior leads to ever-decreasing levels of activity until Deconditioning Syndrome[212] develops, worsening pain, increasing fatigue and decreasing functioning. Avoiding pain becomes a learned response leading to a self-perpetuating cycle causing decline in the musculoskeletal, cardiovascular and nervous systems.[213] Fear of pain, harm and re-injury are major predictors of whether acute pain becomes chronic,[214] and whether someone files for disability or continues to work. Chronic pain patients will have pain whether they do nothing, or are active. For us, pain with activity does not indicate harm.

Psychologist, pain doctor and physical therapist will be the core of your team.

Have Scalpel, Will Travel

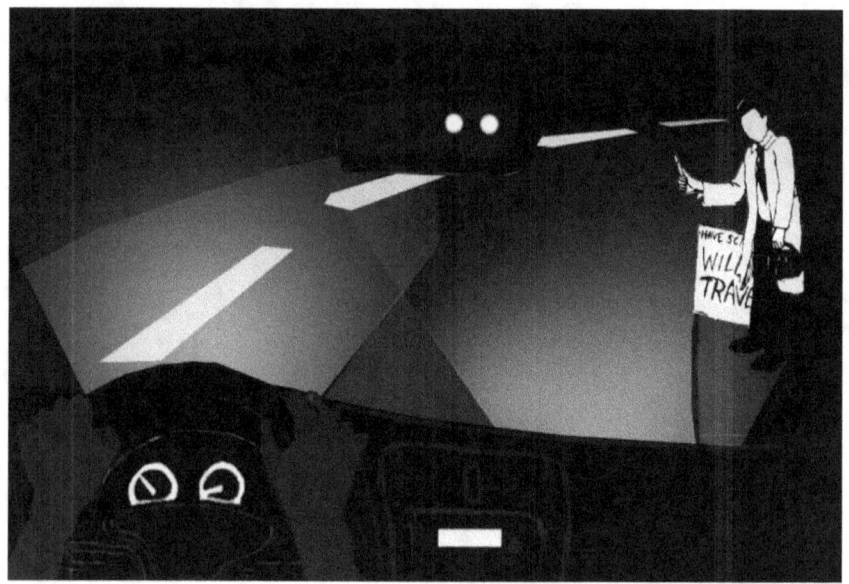

When the pill and needle fail, we turn to the knife. We are a surgery-crazed society. The C-section rate for expectant mothers in 1965 was 5%, today it's 33%.[215] Each specialty is bisected into a medical and surgical component: neurology/neurosurgery; cardiology/cardiac surgery; gastroenterology/general surgery; and pulmonology/thoracic surgery. The push to operate comes from all sides: patients want quick fixes, hospitals want higher profits, and for surgeons, this is business. And business is good.

Doctors chased the pain around my body with needles and burning probes, using hazy x-rays as a guide. Every shadow became the pain generator; and in such pain, who'd say no to a promised cure? Soon the pain will be gone, I was promised, soon. I drank the Kool-Aid, cognitive dissonance set in and I proceeded again and again (and again and again). I write this chapter with purpose: to deter a rush to surgery, and to educate you on the one thing surgeons don't discuss—the evidence.

Private Versus Academic Hospitals

The informed get better treatment, so learn the subtleties of your disease and how health care works. During my career I was surprised how often patients didn't know common-sense things, like the difference between inpatient and outpatient. Here are the basics.

Private hospitals treat everyday problems, like removing an appendix or gallbladder, better than academic hospitals. They are factories: they do a few things well, and focus on volume. Most surgeries are routine, and these cogs fit well into the private hospital machine. There are no residents learning their trade, and your surgeon will have done the operation hundreds of times. Private hospitals function in a capital market, competing for your patronage with radio ads. With a focus on efficiency, they make you better, quickly, and get you home, quickly. And during your stay, there's an effort to keep you comfortable: the rooms, cafeteria, food and staff will be noticeably nicer.

If you have a rare diagnosis—are an oddly shaped cog—you fit better into the academic hospital. Unlike a factory, an academic hospital is an expert craftsmen creating a product from a blueprint. They juggle three competing duties—patient care, research and teaching—and attract inquisitive doctors who focus on esoteric diseases. And like attracts like: a hospital well-known for brain surgery attracts the best brain surgeons. Most are not-for-profit, pouring their capital into this triple duty instead of advertising. Not every academic center excels in each discipline; there are gaping holes you want to avoid.

Johns Hopkins and Stanford are known for pain management because they have in-patient chronic pain services to admit patients for weeks at a time. Many enter inpatient pain programs undiagnosed, receive prolonged attention from different disciplines, and leave correctly diagnosed. But getting admitted to an inpatient pain program is difficult, because the costs are great and the spaces few.

Academic hospitals are also where you enroll in trials of new medications or procedures. Because they don't compete with private hospitals, they cater less to aesthetics: your hospital room will need painting, the cafeteria will have bland food and the attitude will be found wanting. You'll be woken early morning by a medical student followed an hour later by a resident, then a third time by an attending physician (all before 6 AM).

The Four Stages of Surgery

We must tiptoe towards the O.R., otherwise we'll be churned through the sausage factory, emerging pulverized and unrecognizable. Scars from the scalpel remind us of each failure—and here we are, still in pain. If this has already happened, it's okay, you did nothing wrong; there was no more educated patient that entered the sausage factory than I. Anesthesiologists are risk averse by nature, and with back surgeries even more so, because we've anesthetized patients for their fourth, fifth and twentieth back surgeries. But then my pain began, my thinking changed, and I tried and failed repeatedly too.

There are four stages to recognize with regard to any surgical procedure.

Stage 1: Anticipation

No matter how excited your physician is to find the cause of your pain, don't join him in this excitement. The key to rewarding medical results, like happiness, is low expectations. After my first two failed back fusions, the doctors that followed loved having me as a patient because I'd tell them up front, "I consider a pain reduction of 10% a great success." I saw the weight lift off their shoulders as I expressed these expectations—the goal they were kicking the soccer ball into just doubled in size. And when the procedure did fail, they still had vigor to try something different, so at-ease I made them feel.

Stage 2: Surgery hurts

Knowing anxiety worsens pain, and pain worsens anxiety, take steps to calm yourself beforehand. Request sedation before or during your procedure: 1 mg of Versed offers wonders in the way of relaxation. Every procedure suite has the option of sedation, but this means the facility has to recover you after the procedure, taking time and money. I've witnessed all procedures done with local anesthesia without sedation, with mild sedation or with full general anesthesia. Because the average patient tolerates a procedure without sedation doesn't mean you will, since chronic pain causes hyper-sensitivity to ordinarily tolerable pain. Ask your doctor specifically, and he'll agree (because he doesn't have to recover you, the nurses do). If you have a reluctant physician, pre-medicate yourself at home with your own supply of anti-anxiety medications.

Stage 3: Failure

Preserve the bond with your physician, despite failure. The doctor will be proud of the surgery, his art, and insulted when you report it didn't work. Reassuring him that failure is okay—was even expected—will strengthen this bond. Understand human psychology, that we all want to feel successful, and respect it. Being unbearably negative will cause your surgeon to throw his hands up in despair, say the pain is in your head, and blame you for the failure. Know exactly what you will say when the procedure fails.

Stage 4: Now what?

Give the procedure time to work. Treating chronic pain is like running a marathon; sprinting at any stage will decrease your finishing time—the pain relief success rate. Injected steroids provide immediate relief, followed by weeks of no relief, then a resurgence of pain relief. A quick second procedure will confuse the results of the first. Keep a pain diary, follow-up with your physician and don't just disappear. Ask if his needle was in the correct space? Has a radiologist looked at the films? When will he consider the next step? Tiptoe.

Evidence-Based Medicine

What works and what doesn't, and why are things proven not to work still being done? I presented the medical evidence for OA already, so here I present the surgical options for this diagnosis.

The Arthroscopic Placebo

One treatment for OA is arthroscopic surgery of the knee; a scope is inserted into the knee and the surgeon cuts away bits of cartilage (debridement) and washes out the knee (lavage). A subset of orthopedic surgeons practice this surgery, and grabbed more real estate by expanding to the shoulder.

A 2002 *New England Journal of Medicine* study[216] randomized patients into three groups which were all put under anesthesia and received incisions in the knee. One-third of the patients received the standard debridement of cartilage, the second third received lavage of the knee joint and the third group had their incisions sewn back up without any intervention (sham surgery). One surgeon—likely now hated, but bless him—performed all the operations, and all patients and evaluators were blinded to which treatment they received. Follow-up results at one and two years post-op revealed no advantage in pain control of the standard surgical debridement over the placebo group. Gulp.

However science being science, results must be reproduced. A 2008 follow-up study,[217] again in the prestigious *New England Journal of Medicine*, randomized two groups of similar patients to the surgical arthroscopic debridement versus physical therapy without surgery. The results revealed no improvement in pain of the surgical group compared to the intensive physical therapy group. Double gulp.

The studies were denounced by arthroscopic orthopedic surgeons (obviously), but the data invalidates a operation from which an entire subspecialty of surgery subsists. Medicare stopped reimbursing for the operation, but through word-play surgeons are still be reimbursed when a diagnosis with a different name is used (e.g. knee pain NOS). So the operation persists.[218] How can this be? Well, hospitals make money off the procedure and have bargaining power with insurance companies (reimburse for all our procedures or we'll stop accepting your insurance hospital-wide). Money buys influence. But it begs the question, has anyone looked into the benefits of arthroscopic surgery of the shoulder? Many operations proved worthless continue to be performed, as this article reveals.[219]

Back Pain Evidence

Eighty percent of humans will, at some point in their lives, experience low back pain. 60% experienced back pain within the last year, and 80%-90% of these pain episodes recover within six weeks without any treatment.[220] Sciatica occurs when a disc in the back bulges, compressing the nerves that go into the leg, causing shooting pain (*radiculopathy*). The natural course of untreated sciatica is that the pain will resolve within eight weeks for the majority of patients.[221, 222]

Despite this, the trend is still quick referral of these patients to spine surgeons for both sciatica and low back pain without the requisite tincture of time or conservative therapy. A RCT[223] in 1983(!) showed that when surgery was compared to conservative care in patients with disc herniation, the outcome of surgery was superior at the one-year follow-up. This became a "landmark study" within the spine surgery community and led to a massive rise in spine operations. Spinal fusions continued to soar between 1997 and 2008, increasing Medicare costs from $343 million to $2.24 billion, a 400% increase after adjustment for inflation.[224] The complexity and number of implants has also skyrocketed, as one surgeon put it, "you can easily put $30,000 worth of hardware into a patient during a fusion surgery."[225] The hardware being implanted is often manufactured by a company the surgeon partially owns. The more implants used, the better the manufacturer does, and the better the manufacturer does, the better the partial owner (the surgeon) does. Recent articles in the *Wall Street Journal* entitled "Taking Double Cut, Surgeons Implant Their Own Devices" and "Top Spine Surgeons Reap Royalties, Medicare Bounty" have exposed this. I had screws, rods and replacement discs implanted in me; I wonder if my surgeon part-owned the company that made them? A conflict of interest like this should be disclosed to patients.

We are amidst a great epidemic of increasing back pain and disc herniations; or, less dramatically, we are in the midst of an epidemic of too early surgical treatment, along with an unnecessary increasing complexity of surgeries (led by the financial incentives for surgeons to increase the use of hardware). Things are getting out of control and the question needs to be asked: what does the evidence show? Not the evidence from the "landmark study" in 1983, but more recent up-to-date studies. Spine surgeons in private practice will not be current with the recent literature. Surgeons at academic centers are more likely to know the up-to-date literature.

A *New England Journal of Medicine* article[226] in 2007 randomized patients with sciatica to either early surgical disc removal or conservative therapy. Patients randomized to undergo surgery had quicker relief of pain, but at one year's time, the two groups were identical. Is waiting a year with pain worth avoiding a back surgery? A repeat study[227] yielded similar results: surgery "offered only modest short-term benefits in patients with sciatica due to disc extrusion" when compared to conservative non-operative treatment.

A *JAMA* study[228] looking back through medical charts compared trends of older patients undergoing surgery for spinal stenosis. The results showed that between 2002 and 2007, the invasiveness of surgeries increased even though the data showed more complex surgeries were associated with an increased risk of major complications, 30-day mortality and resource use.

A study[229] examining MRIs of the spine showed a high prevalence of disk bulges and protrusions in people without back pain, leading the authors to conclude, "the discovery by MRI of bulges or protrusions in people with low back pain may frequently be coincidental." If we all have disc bulges and disc herniations, pain and non-pain populations alike, how can they be identified as pain generators?

Even a 1987 review article four years after the landmark study recognized the trend, "Disc surgery has survived the test of time for half a century because at least 70–80 percent of carefully accepted patients obtain relief. Such dramatic surgical successes unfortunately only apply to approximately 1 percent of patients with low-back disorders."[230] The results show the best course of treatment for sciatica, barring red flags like bowel or bladder involvement, is to let natural recovery occur. Patients will have the same pain and disability level at one year's time whether they have surgery or allow natural healing.

Anesthesia

Anesthesia revolutionized surgery. Before ether was discovered in 1842, surgeries had to be "swift of hand." A basic understanding of anesthesia helps to understand the transmission of pain, and thus its treatment, to allay the fears for the inevitable surgeries you'll undergo. In common parlance, anesthesia means falling asleep so you don't feel an operation. The medical definition of anesthesia has four components:

- Anesthesia: a state of unconsciousness.
- Analgesia: pain relief.
- Amnesia: no recall or memory of the events.
- Immobility: rendering a patient immobile during an operation.

Anesthesia is a state of unconsciousness separate from analgesia, pain relief. Newer versions of inhaled ether and chloroform render a patient unconscious; yet a scalpel cutting through the skin of an unconscious patient will still provoke a pain response, observed as a rise in heart rate and blood pressure. And if the surgeon continues to cut, and the anesthesiologist keeps the patient "only unconscious," eventually the patient will have a heart attack and die. The body feels pain without awareness, thus the need for analgesia.

Analgesia is the blockage of pain transmission to the brain, and is achieved with either local anesthesia or intravenous opioids. This one component of the four can stand alone, and does stand alone in the example of spinal or epidural anesthesia where sensation from the chest to the toes is blocked and the patient is kept awake and conversant during the operation (drapes blocking their view). If the surgery is on the arm or leg, anesthesiologists perform nerve blocks of this extremity, gaining the advantage of avoiding general anesthesia and opioids. Some brain tumor removals are done with the patient wide awake, because brain tissue has no pain receptors; so a patient's ability to speak and respond can be tested throughout the surgery if the operation is near a part of the brain involved in speaking or hearing.

Amnesia is caused by intravenous benzodiazepines, stronger versions of Valium or Xanax, which cause powerful memory loss and are given as a backstop, to cover fragments of memory a patient remembers. They cause both anterograde amnesia (when you can't make new memories from the point after the drug is given) as well as retrograde amnesia (memories already made are wiped out). Each time I had a back surgery I'd forget the day after surgery, as well as driving to the hospital the day of surgery.

The final component of anesthesia is *immobility*. You can render a patient unconscious, amnestic and pain free, but when the scalpel cuts through muscle it will jump and react to the blade. This is where muscle relaxant drugs come in; derivatives of curare, a plant extract Native Americans put on arrowheads to paralyze their prey. These agents block the transmission between nerve and muscle, allowing the surgeon to move away the normally tense and reactive muscles. But it also blocks the muscles used to breath, so patients under anesthesia need to have a breathing tube put in so their breathing can be taken over (intubation).

The anesthesiologist juggles each of these four balls during surgery to ensure the perfect operating conditions for the surgeon, and the perfect pain-free state for the patient. Too much or too little of any of the four can result in problems. Too little *anesthesia* (unconsciousness) and the patient will experience recall from the surgery; too much and they will be slow to wake up. To little *analgesia* (pain relief) and the patient's heart rate and blood pressure will skyrocket; too much opioid and the patient will not breath upon waking. Too little *amnesia* is a problem only if your unconsciousness fails; too much of the amnestic drugs wipes out a whole week of time. Too little *muscle relaxation* and the muscles jump and move to incision; too much and the patient can't move when they emerge from anesthesia. The nightmare disaster of the anesthesia gas running out, allowing consciousness to return, but being unable to move because of the muscle relaxants in your system occurs but a handful of times across the entire US and isn't something to worry about. Of these four elements analgesia—pain relief—is the most important. If a patient does not experience any pain, then unconsciousness, amnesia, and immobility are helpful, but secondary.

Surgery #2

Surgery #1 was a lumbar fusion of the bottom two vertebral levels. Six months later the pain was worse. A "flexion-extension x-ray" was done: I bent forward and had an x-ray snapped, and then bent backwards and had another. Comparing these films showed the joint was still moving—not fused!

We couldn't even determine if facet syndrome was the correct diagnosis, because the joints were still moving. Five months later, across the country on the other coast, a private surgeon rolled me into another operating room to "re-do" the first operation properly (surgery #2).

I will continue this thread in the next chapter, but want to highlight the "next step" trap I fell into. No one expects an MRI will hurt them, but it led to an invasive and painful discogram. The theory of lidocaine injections in my back led to one surgery, complications during hospitalization, and then another surgery. In a doctor's mind, any positive or indeterminate result needs further work-up, which leads to more next steps and further work-up. Before you know it you'll have had two back operations for the wrong diagnosis. Ask yourself and your doctor, "What will we do if this test is positive?"

Doctors get paid to operate: buyer beware.

What If This is As Good As It Gets?

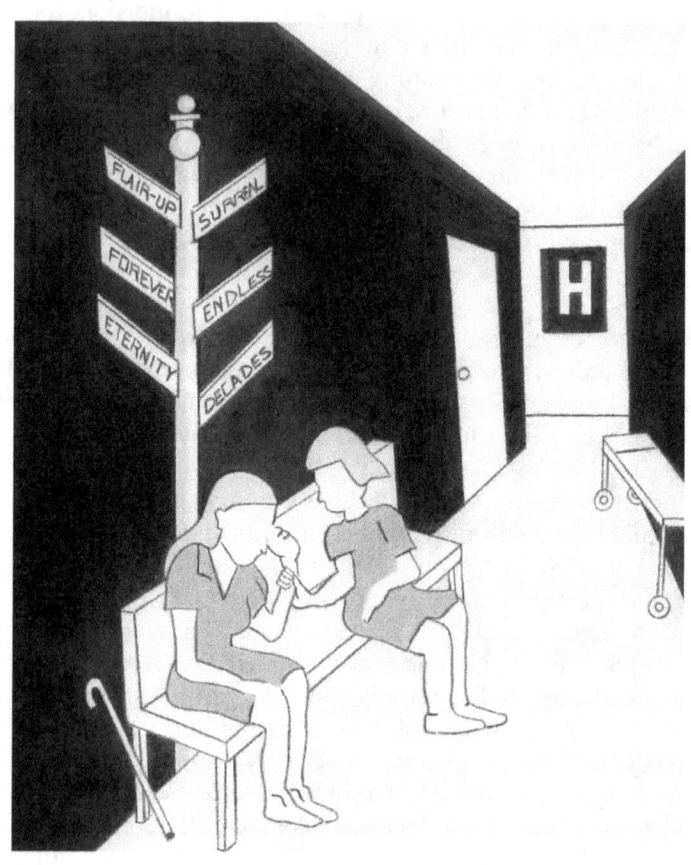

"It is not the strongest species that survive, nor the most intelligent, but the ones most responsive to change."

—Charles Darwin

I sat in my surgeon's waiting room nine months after my second spine operation—cane in each hand, rigid back brace, zero pain relief. A Japanese woman moved to a seat beside me, and asked my story. I told her. She surprised me with a similar tale: nine months post-op and still in pain. What she said next prompted this chapter. She gripped my forearm, faced me and said, "I'm so scared. What if we never get better?"

Her terror stunned me. It was dawning on her that this is it, *as good as it gets*, as Jack Nicholson said to a psychiatry waiting room in the movie of the same name. I put my arm around her and said, "It'll be all right." Her words turned back time; two years earlier I was as spooked as she was. Once equally afraid, I had moved past the fear, and was serene that day in my surgeon's office. How had I transitioned?

"Time heals all wounds" is false, for it hasn't healed my burning groin and leg pain; but it has chipped away at the worry that pain brings. Few situations arise that I haven't already encountered, overcome, and survived. Finagling and figuring through a life with pain inculcated in me an experienced calm. How to get groceries and cook with such pain? How to be happy with such pain? How to have sex with such pain? How to? How to? These questions were answered for me over the years. For it is no longer what if? or how to? It is.

Surgery #3

After a year of physical therapy to strengthen the muscles of my pelvis and hip, my SI joint continued "going out" (dislocating) 1-3 times a day. I was able to lie flat, pull knee to chest and push my leg out, relocating my hip to its proper position and correcting the leg length discrepancy. To keep the dislocations down I curtailed my physical activities: I stopped walking up hills, stairs or carrying anything heavier than a quart of milk. I stopped improving. Janelle had taught me everything she knew about the SI joint, and still wanted me to wait for the ligaments to tighten. But after a year, I gave up on this and started looking for a proper fix.

The SI joint moves only a few millimeters, and auto-fuses in elderly men without them even knowing it. I wanted mine fixed in place, despite the protestations of my primary care doctor, pain specialist and Janelle. I began a nationwide search for a surgeon to cement this joint. A third spine surgery, after two wrecks, scared me too; but I was an invalid with a loosey-goosey hip. It was worth the risk.

I read every article written on SI joint fusion and made a (very short) list of surgeons who specialized in this operation. The surgical evidence gave me pause. It was horrible. My surgeon in Los Angeles told me he had done the operations a "handful of times," but I wanted someone who only did it. He said the rarity of the diagnosis made it unlikely anyone would specialize in it, but he gave me two names on the west coast who he'd have operate on him if he needed this surgery. A starting point.

My care providers formed a brick wall of resistance, so I didn't tell my parents what I was planning. The only person in my family who knew was my uncle in England, also an orthopedic surgeon, who gave me the same answer: the results are poor, don't do it. I had been living part time with my parents and part time out of state, but moved permanently away to keep this secret. The two west coast surgeons evaluated me, and said I was a candidate for the surgery. They had each performed the surgery at least 50 times, but their practices were still primarily lumbar fusions. I decided to move further up the food chain, and asked each of them who they'd have operate on them if they needed this operation. I expected them to name each other, but they didn't. They both pointed to the name of one doctor in Atlanta, familiar to me because of his many publications on SI fusion surgery.

Off to Georgia I went. He was French and spoke heavily accented English, but was a neurosurgeon and not an orthopedic surgeon, which I liked (because they're just more intelligent people). The morning of my appointment I carried my suitcase up and down the stairs of my hotel 15 times, causing my hip to malrotate horribly. I limped to see him in intense pain—my groin, thighs and hips aflame. I wanted to relocate my hip bone, but resisted, and was glad I didn't because the first thing he checked for was for a leg length discrepancy. I lay flat on his examining table, one foot was six inches longer than the other. "See," I said as I rotated it back in front of him. He was impressed with this display.

He wanted to do a lidocaine injection into the SI joint to see if it relived my pain. He set up the appointment for that afternoon (75% of his patients were from out of state, so he made same-day procedure appointments). I went to the flouroscopy suite and he injected my SI joint up and down with lidocaine. "Any pain relief?" he asked. No. Zero. But my pain was only when my hip was subluxed, which I had corrected earlier that morning. He said that he was tentative to operate on me without improvement in pain from the injection. He described the operation: he'd put two screws through my hip bone into my butt bone (sacrum) under x-ray guidance, then cut open the joint and pack it with soft bone, which would solidify over the weeks to permanently fuse the joint.

I too was afraid of another operation, any operation. I was in the exact situation as before my first surgery; we were convinced of the diagnosis, knew the needed fix, but some middling procedure that should have confirmed everything failed. I lunged ahead last time, to disaster. I asked for "an elegant solution," an in-between step to further prove the diagnosis without cutting me open. He proposed a halfway step, putting only the screws in under x-ray guidance without an incision, to see if I achieved relief.

If I did, he'd follow-up with the second half of the surgery at a later date. This way it was minimally invasive and a test to see if the SI joint was the pain generator. (I liked his healthy skepticism of the diagnosis that I was now convinced of.) I got dressed, and as I was leaving I asked him, "How many times have you done this surgery?"

"This is the only operation I do. I haven't done a lumbar fusion in five years."

And with that I made up my mind to have the operation. I returned home and ran all by my pain specialist, primary care doctor and Janelle. They were aghast, all against it. "Why is the evidence so bad?" they countered. This was a fair question, so I called Atlanta and passed the query along.

"The evidence is bad because surgeons just fuse the joint in whatever position it's in, without realigning it. The key is to line up the joint correctly with fluoroscopy, so all the crannies-and-nooks are aligned, and then put the screws in." He told me his data wasn't bad; the RCTs he had performed showed excellent results.

I went over every study he had published later that evening, as crannies-and-nooks went through my head. He was correct. His trials had good results after fusion. Central was understanding that there are six different positions the SI joint can be in, and aligning these three axis before fusing the joint is the step surgeons are ignorant to. They fuse the joint with either a *rotation*, *upslip* or *flair*. I called and scheduled the surgery.

My pain took me to five states for second, third, even tenth opinions, but found a remedy in a small hospital in the suburbs of Atlanta, Georgia. I searched for the best of the best, and knew I'd found him when he said, "That's the only operation I do."

Travel to find the best of the best.

Alternative Treatments

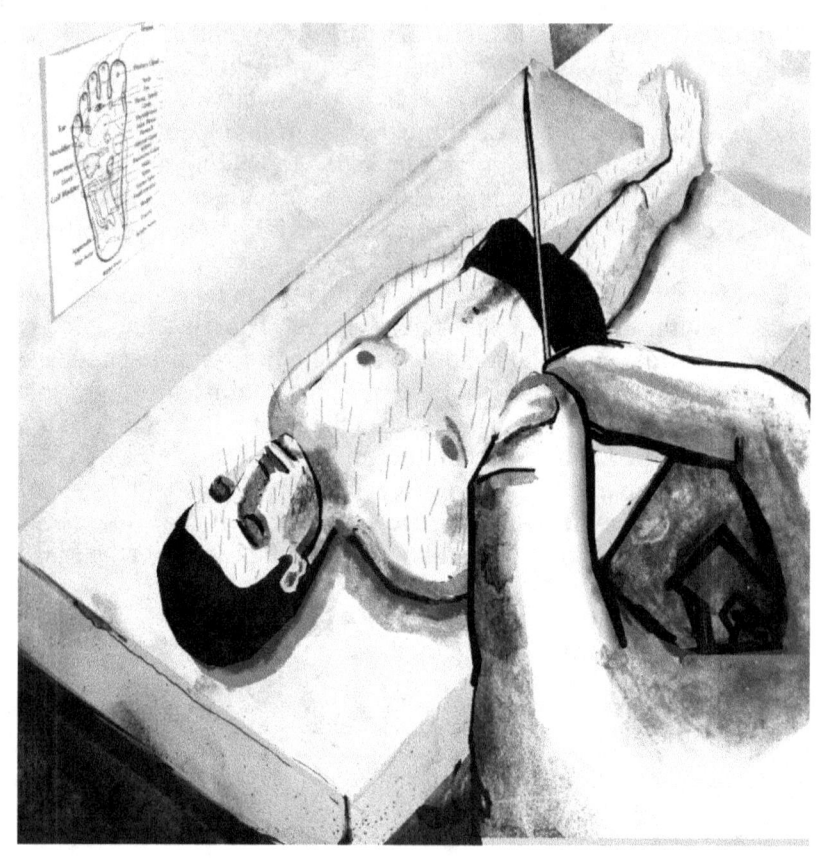

"The inappropriate treatment of pain includes non-treatment, under-treatment, over-treatment and the continued use of ineffective treatments."

—Federation of State Medical Boards

Few of us will find a silver bullet cure, and those who do, me for instance, will see the silver rust as the pain continues despite the fix. The more valuable "procedure" is to learn to cope, whether that's through acceptance, a medication or one of these boutique offerings. There is a land between "procedure" and "operation" of options unadvertised to patients or internists. Two examples are Nerve Stimulation and Spinal Drug Delivery: these palliative measures exist in a purgatory, sometimes performed in procedure rooms with local anesthesia and sedation, other times in operating rooms under general anesthesia.

Nerve Stimulation

Jerry Lewis used the pratfall as his shtick, tripping, running into walls and falling on his face for laughs. He had it perfected; but an estimated 1,900 falls later, he developed back pain unresponsive to surgery or opioids. He had a spinal cord stimulator implanted, which he described on an episode of Larry King Live (it's worth watching this episode on the web), which replaced pain with a "buzzing" sensation.

Recall the gate control theory of pain: nerves pass through a gate to reach the spinal cord and deliver their data (pain, touch, temperature or vibration). Stub a toe and you'll squeeze it, clogging the gate with "touch signals" to prevent pain signals from reaching the brain. Nerve stimulation adopts this theory: sending electricity along a nerve is akin to continually squeezing your toe, flooding the gate with "other signals" to prevent the pain signals from passing. This led to the spinal cord stimulator (SCS) and peripheral nerve stimulator (PNS), devices implanted by pain specialists and some neurosurgeons at major medical centers. More invasive than the typical back injection, but less invasive than back surgery, the SCS is supported by good evidence and covered by insurance (because it's cheaper than surgery).

Before a SCS is implanted there is a trial: an epidural is performed and a wire is threaded alongside the at-fault-nerve. It's then stimulated with electricity, and re-positioned, until buzzing replaces pain. The voltage is adjusted, deluging the "gate" with electricity until no pain signals pass. Pain is replaced with non-painful buzzing. You are sent home with the wire in place connected to a control box for two days to evaluate the pain relief. If 50% relief is achieved, you go to the OR (or procedure suite) and have the control box implanted under your skin. An external remote control allows you to still adjust the voltage as your pain dictates.

A RCT[231] found the SCS more effective than reoperation in patients with *failed back syndrome* who had greater leg than back pain. Patients randomized to receive the SCS used less opioids and had more functional improvement than those reoperated on. Meta-analysis, a study of studies, revealed 59% of patients treated with a SCS had at least 50% pain relief, improved functioning and reduced opioid use.[232] For the diagnosis CRPS, multiple studies[233] found spinal cord stimulation effective.

The risks are infection and movement of the wire (lead migration) which happens 3%[234] of the time. The advantages are that it's reversible and there's a trial before implantation. Performed for failed back syndrome and peripheral nerves gone mad (complex regional pain syndrome), there is also evidence for its use in migraines,[235] cancer pain, peripheral vascular disease, ischemic chest pain,[236] shingles, burns, nerve trauma and any peripheral nerve pain. There is literature for each diagnosis, so do your homework before taking this step, and find a practitioner who implants these daily, if not exclusively.

But be skeptical of any procedure, especially one touting 50% pain relief. SCS and PNS have few studies, and none of the highest quality because administering a placebo is impossible. It's also a trendy field of medicine, further decreasing the validity of the findings. Studies do show that it's effective and reversible, moving it down the ladder of options, compared to irreversible surgery or opioid eating.

The True "Mainline"

Tablets are given PO (per oral) or PR (per rectum), but liquid medications have many delivery options. The slowest route is subcutaneous (SQ), which takes the longest to take effect, but also lasts the longest (diabetics inject insulin SQ to last throughout the day). Intramuscular injections (IM) take effect faster because muscles are vascularized, and a depot of medication resides in the muscle for hours, prolonging its effect. IM injections take effect faster than SQ, but don't last as long. Intravenous (IV) is the most familiar route, which immediately enters the bloodstream, but also leaves quickly as it's metabolized. Post-op patients receive both IV and IM opioids: the IV dose has an immediate effect, while the IM dose is released over 6-8 hours.

Pain medications work when they reach a nerve receptor. Two routes of administration are faster than IV, because they place the medication directly onto the nerve: epidural and intrathecal. Pain is transmitted through nerves, and the density of receptors increase as you move closer to the spinal cord and brain. PO, IV and IM opioids have to work their way through the blood stream before reaching a nerve's pain receptor, so have a slower and less powerful pain relieving effect (*analgesic effect*).

The spinal cord floats freely in fluid (*CSF*), which is enclosed by three layers of ligaments (*meninges*), and then by the bones of the back (*vertebrae*). The epidural space is outside the third ligament, the dura, thus its name "epi-dural." The spinal nerves branch off the spinal cord, and pass through the liquid zone called the intrathecal space, and exit through the epidural space on their way to the periphery. Pain medications placed in the epidural space have a stronger effect than intravenous (IV) opioids because they are deposited directly onto nerves as they branch off the spinal cord; and opioids injected into the fluid zone (*intrathecally*) have the strongest effect of all because they bathe the spinal cord itself.

When a laboring woman receives an "epidural," a small tube (catheter) is left in place to continuously administer a lidocaine/opioid mixture. When a chronic pain patient receives an "epidural," it's a one-time injection without a wire left behind.

But instead of stopping outside the three layers of meninges, a epidural needle can pass into the fluid buffeting the spinal cord (*the intrathecal space*). The needle can't contact the spinal cord because it ends at the L1/L2 level and the needle is inserted lower at the L4/L5 level. Medication injected intrathecally floats upwards and bathes the spinal cord from the base of the spine up to the brainstem; a powerful route of administration, and the true "mainline" (don't tell heroin addicts).

Spinal anesthesia is performed by injecting local anesthetic into this space, which causes numbness from toes to mid-chest. Opioids have a greater analgesic effect the closer they get to the spinal cord; so, less opioids are needed to attain pain relief. Here's a conversion formula:

$$\frac{100\text{mg morphine}}{\text{given as a pill}} = 10\text{mg IV} = \frac{1\text{mg}}{\text{epidurally}} = \frac{0.1\text{mg}}{\text{intrathecally}}$$

The epidural of a laboring woman exits the skin and connects to a machine administering the opioid/lidocaine mixture. This apparatus has been miniaturized and internalized, and is now available to chronic pain patients. The wire is placed in the epidural or intrathecal space and connected to an implanted box holding a reservoir of medication. The dose is given continuously and controlled with an external remote; refilling the medication requires poking a needle through the skin into the reservoir. Initially developed for cancer patients on high dose opioids, this implanted drug delivery system is available to patients with CNMP.

The opioid is released continuously, avoiding the highs and lows of oral dosing, and removing the hassle of obtaining and filling prescriptions. The downsides are the same as for opioids—respiratory depression, itching, constipation, nausea, tolerance—along with machine malfunction and the risk of the box being implanted (the infection rate is 2%).[237]

Studies[238] have proven the safety and efficacy of medications delivered in this fashion, neuraxially, for those who choose the opioid path (not I). One patient I saw with an implanted epidural drug delivery system stands out: he had CRPS of the leg, and the slightest touch caused pain. His epidural pump contained only local anesthetic and was activated one hour before physical therapy. The anesthetic numbed his leg, allowing it to be desensitized with massage, as well as having his toe nails cut. It was a novel use of an implanted pump, permitting physical therapy that would have been otherwise impossible.

Complementary Alternative Medicine (CAM)

Acupuncture, biofeedback, chiropractic manipulation, herbal medicine, hypnotherapy, massage, osteopathy and relaxation therapy all complement mainstream medicine; they are grouped under the category Complementary Alternative Medicine (or CAM). Looking for RCTs and systematic reviews for the effectiveness of CAM revealed a dearth of high quality evidence. The few RCTs showing a positive effect have not been successfully replicated by other investigators.

The following diagnoses have proven CAM treatments:

- Migraine: Biofeedback and relaxation training.[239]
- Osteo-arthritis: acupuncture[240], PhytodolorTM[241] and S-adenosylmethionine.[242]
- Rheumatoid-arthritis: Fasting, vegetarian diet[243], fish oil[244] and tai chi.[245]
- Fibromyalgia: Exercise.
- Post-operative pain: Hypnotherapy[246] and TENS.[247]

While advertised as natural, CAM has been associated with adverse effects[248]: puncture of vital organs with acupuncture, arterial damage with chiropractic manipulation (including documented deaths) and toxicity with herbal medicine.

Peripheral Nerve and Plexus Blocks

After nerves branch off the spine cord, they pass through the fluid zone, three ligaments, the bones of the back and then run to the periphery. If you block these nerves with lidocaine, there will be numbness downstream (*distal*) from the point of injection. Nerves in the periphery are surrounded by tissue and not bone, so live x-ray (*fluoroscopy*) can't be used to guide the needle as it is with the spine. Peripheral nerves are located in two ways. The first is a field block: the doctor knows anatomically where the nerve runs, and injects lidocaine in a range to spread and hit the nerve. The second way is with a nerve stimulator, which pulses electricity through a needle that is advanced toward the nerve. Once the needle is close, the current will run through the nerve to the muscle, causing it to contract rhythmically. The electricity is turned down, the needle is advanced closer to the nerve, then the lidocaine is injected.

A nerve can be injected at multiple points along its path: a nerve to the leg will exit the spinal cord and pass through the epidural space, where the epidural injection (the "shotgun" blast) can access it. It then leaves the epidural space and divides as it leaves the vertebral bones of the back, where each spinal nerve can be injected (a "sniper shot"), or the facet joints that allow the back to move can be injected. As the nerve moves to the periphery it can be injected in the groin (femoral nerve), the thigh (sciatic nerve), behind the knee (popliteal nerve) or at the ankle.

Hospitals that specialize in orthopedic surgery use nerve blocks and sedation, not general anesthesia, for surgery. The advantage is that the block lasts for a day, providing pain relief without opioids. Sometimes they also leave a wire (*catheter*) on a peripheral nerve to continually pump lidocaine as they do with epidurals.

The three most common peripheral nerves injected for chronic pain are the pudendal nerve (for pelvic pain), the occipital nerve (for tension headaches caused by tight muscles) and an entrapped lateral femoral cutaneous nerve (for a condition called meralgia paraesthetica).

The Pain Ladder

With chronic pain, our presentation-diagnosis-treatment is indefinite, and there are few statistical models directing what to do when. You're left with your expert opinion medicine, which will differ from doctor to doctor. In a later chapter I present a "pain menu;" but a menu infers a choosing, and if the pain is severe you'll skip the appetizers—physical therapy, psychotherapy, time—and jump to the main course, surgery.

A "pain ladder" is a better term.[249] Start on the first rung and slowly climb, adding treatments to those already in effect, instead of starting one and stopping another. Move methodically higher, beginning with lower echelon drugs versus higher echelon drugs (Vicodin before Oxycontin), less invasive procedures over more invasive (steroid injections before nerve burning) and less invasive operations over more invasive (micro-discectomy over spinal fusion). The ladder won't fall away from the house, so take your time climbing higher.

Surgery #4

The screws the surgeon twisted through my hip bone held it in place. The subluxations and leg length discrepancy stopped, but the "feeling" of instability continued. And, of course, the pain continued, albeit at a lower $4/10$ level. I was terrified of putting any weight on the hip with the screws through it, in case it caused them to dislodge or "back out," as the surgeon said happens 1% of the time. I clung to both canes, wore my SI belt tight and didn't dare do any PT. After a year, I returned to see my French neurosurgeon.

He looked at the film and said the screws were in position, and he was pleased the dislocations had stopped. But I begged for step 2, the second half of the surgery. He began describing it to me. It included making an incision over the SI joint to pack it full of soft bone that would turn solid and fuse the joint. But this entailed cutting the muscles and ligaments holding the hip in place, something he didn't like doing.

I didn't like the sound of that either, but I needed more stability. "Isn't there any other option?" I asked. He paused, contemplating his words, then told me there was. An experimental approach to access the SI joint that he had done only a few times, but that he felt was revolutionary and perfect for me. Imagine 2 bananas lying side by side, one the hip bone and one the sacrum. The typical surgeon makes an incision over the gap between the two bananas, cutting through the muscles and ligaments holding the bananas together. His new technique was a sideways approach, approaching the gap by tunneling through the body of one of the bananas. He'd cut a hole in my hip right bone, one of the bananas, the size of a golf ball and take the removed bone and shove it into the joint space. This would be done with an incision on the side of my body, and wouldn't cut any ligaments or muscles.

It made sense: Why cut supporting structures when this alternate route is possible? Trying to add stability to a joint by cutting the muscles and ligaments currently stabilizing it seemed mad. Why was this experimental and not the gold standard? His answer was that it's not how other surgeons did the operation, the "standard of care." What if the standard of care was wrong; how do you create a new standard if you can't deviate from the current?

I understood his trepidation operating differently than everyone else; one bad outcome and you're defenseless in a courtroom. He said he would do the operation, but only because I was a physician and could give true "informed consent." Any other patient could claim afterwards they didn't understand the medical lingo and wouldn't have given consent. Let this illustrate to you the importance of setting your physician at-ease for failed medications, procedures and surgeries. It's not their fault any more than the medications' fault for not taking away the pain.

Know your options.

III. Now What?

"He Who Has a Why to Live Can Bear With Any How."

— Friedrich Nietzsche

When is Enough, Enough?

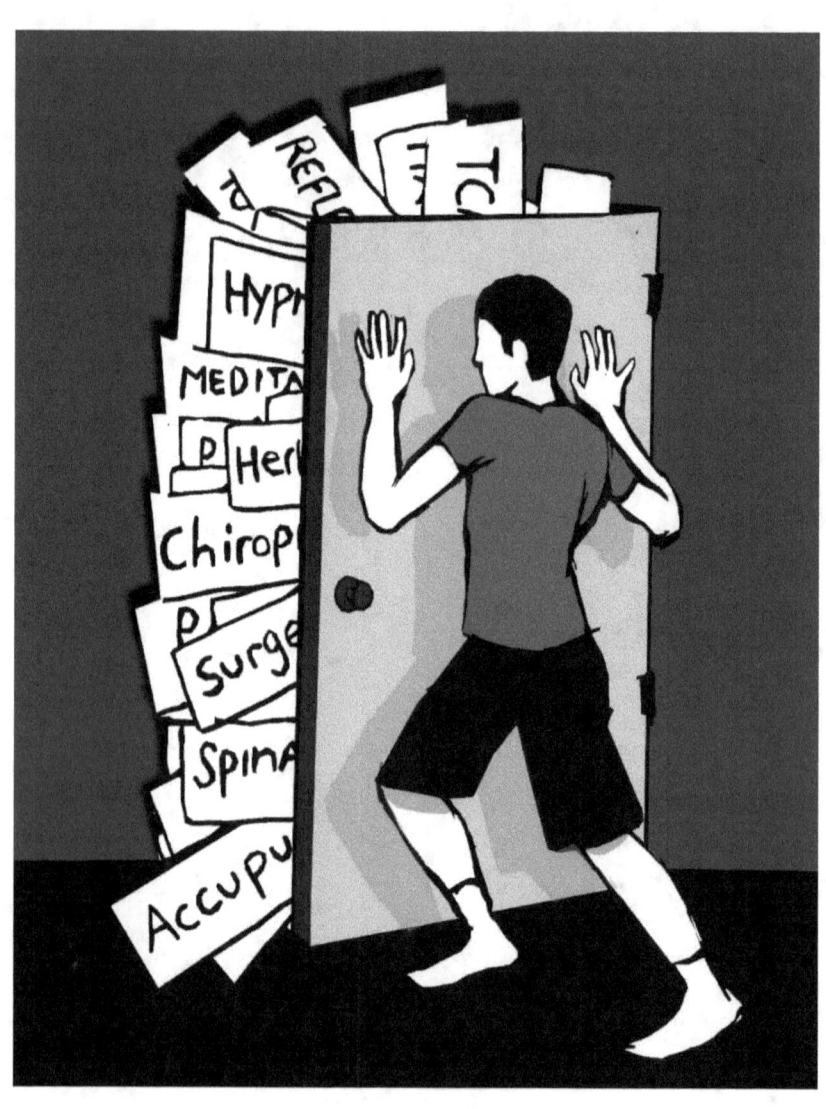

"Out of options, I joined the other no-hopers at Mayo's pain rehabilitation center. There, chronic pain, unlike the acute variety, was treated as a malfunction in perceptions, whether or not an ongoing physical cause had been identified. The brain becomes addicted to dramatizing pain, they said; and the more you feed it, the stronger the addiction. So don't dwell on the pain, and don't try to fix it—no props, no pills. Eventually the mind should go."

—*New York Times*, David Roberts[250]

Accepting Foreverness

The dawning that the pain isn't going to be cured, but managed, is the second step in your progression to acceptance. Recognition will not occur suddenly one day, but slowly over a period of failed diagnoses and treatments. Amid the jumble of procedures, clinics and pharmacies you'll cross a line of awareness that your pain is no longer binary—pain or no pain—but a sliding scale off which you cannot jump.

The first change is definitional: acute becomes chronic. You're re-categorized in computers, insurance companies and medical charts. Only the nomenclature changes, but subtleties of those who read that text will become evident to you in their body language or attitude.

Next you will declare the new definition; the first time you say, "I have chronic pain," it will sound foreign to you. As you repeat it, a sadness sets in for your former self. Allow this. Mourning will ease the transition; you hold onto a thread of hope to return to being pain-free, but that thread thins as the months turn into years, and snaps during your Dark Night.

You wend your way from injury or ailment, to illness. But here we are, ill; not with cancer or lupus, but something just as weighty. I had a tennis injury and referred to the time "before my injury" and "after my injury." Now I allude to the time "before I got sick" and "after I got sick."

The next transition is the hardest; moving from seeking a pain cure, to pain management. There are still treatments and pills to improve your pain; a grease to ease you lower on the slide we call the pain scale. Continue all treatments to their logical endpoints, even as you solidify a new mindset of foreverness. See your doctors, go to appointments, and have procedures or surgeries, if warranted; there's a lot available these days to improve, not cure, pain. Be just as determined to improve your pain as you once were to cure your pain. Hope abounds as new technologies are developed, new trials completed and new medicines synthesized.

When the pain first began you entered a manic phase as you rifled around for a cure; now you know there is no cure, permit a new mania to set in: a shotgun approach, trying everything, to discover what provides *relief.* Here are some of the therapies, practitioners and medications I tried during this second phase of symptom control:

- Massage therapy, biofeedback, myofascial release, chiropractors, Neurontin, Lyrica, acupuncture, psychotherapy, physical therapy, aroma therapy, naturopathic doctors, Chinese medicine.
- Inpatient pain management programs, pain support groups, neuroemotional technique (NET), TENS units, capsaicin cream, sacroiliac belts, back braces, splints of all kinds.
- And then there's prolotherapy, energy therapy, MRI-guided injections, neuroablation techniques, epidural injections, steroid injections.
- And even hypnosis, rheumatologists, peripheral nerve neurosurgeons, orthopedists, and rolfing.

No one can foresee which combination of drug, procedure and therapist will reduce your pain the most. I had a motley crew come to my rescue: Diagnosed by a novice physical therapist, fixed by a French neurosurgeon in Atlanta and reincorporated into life by a social worker in the role of a psychologist.

"Trying everything," as I did, entails risk; I found this out the hard way after two back surgeries for the wrong diagnosis. There are complications, side effects, bad reactions and poor outcomes from any medication, procedure or surgery. So be guided by someone who can ensure a reasonable chance that a certain drug or therapy has a chance of helping you. If something does help, if you have the resources, find the best of that thing. When I was working during this stage, I flew to Baltimore, Los Angeles, San Francisco, South Carolina, and Hawaii until I found what I was looking for in Atlanta: my French neurosurgeon. Run the gamut to convince yourself you've tried everything; you won't be able to reach acceptance, and build a new identity, if there's a glowing injection or procedure that you're sure will help.

The last transition of this step is not one you take, but one taken for you: your doctor will acknowledge your pain is chronic, and that there's little left to help you. This will lead to a confrontation and distancing in your relationship. A heart-to-heart here is necessary; explain you want to reach the same point of acceptance, but there is a line in the sand between a quest for a cure versus symptom management. My words fell flat in this discussion, as might yours. The transition is complete when your physician begins developing coping strategies for dealing with you:

> The physician is forced to devise his or her own strategies for coping with such unrewarding patients. Spending as little time as possible with the patient, referral to another specialist, and simply prescribing narcotic analgesics are common strategies.[251]

When you note this happening, be done with that doctor. Take control, and self-refer to the specialists you want to see. This led me to a physical therapist (who diagnosed me), a surgeon (who fixed me), and a psychologist (who talked me through it all). I had two corrective surgeries, but it was too long after the onset of pain to be curative: the injury was fixed, the illness remains.

My psychologist and I disagreed over the question: When is enough, enough? I accepted there was no cure to my pain, but couldn't accept there wasn't more to palliate my pain. Searching gave me bursts of hope as I stumbled upon new doctors, drugs, and procedures. I knew this hope was a placebo; but what harm is there in taking a sugar pill to feel better? My psychologist countered that the chase took away from experiences in the here and now. My head was buried in a quest and I missed the flowers of spring, the job offer, the relationship, the family and the marrow of being alive. She urged me to skip appointments and go for a walk instead.

You need to make your own decision when enough is enough. For me it was easy as there was nothing left to do that made sense. I pass this wrenching decision to you: do you expand your procedure list by one, or learn a new hobby? Start a new drug, or go out to dinner? Compare these two statements:

"You have to live with the pain"

"You have to accept the pain."

Patients and doctors dread the first, because it indicates failure, finality and a "get out of my clinic because there's nothing left for you here." The second sentence feels different; what does it mean to accept pain? It doesn't sound like an ending, but a beginning—embarking on something new.

The Pain-Time Continuum

Chronic pain slows time.

Well, not really, but it slows the perception of time. But let's begin even simpler.

Novelty slows the perception of time. New experiences erect signposts in the mind which serve as scaffolding for memory. Every happening creates an impression, but the true rebar and concrete of memory is built from fresh events—novelty. The more unique occasions, the more permanent signposts you plant. And the more signposts, the greater that period of time "seems" to last. Look back at a memorable event, like your wedding or any other once-in-a-lifetime event, and that period of time sprawls out in your mind. One memorable weekend will feel like a week, as the new experiences slow time down, broadening the space it takes up in the mind.

This is why childhood seems to "last" longer than adulthood, because the continual newness raises more banners to look back at. This happens to a couple with a new baby; time slows down because of all the firsts: the first poop, the first step, the first word and the first day at school. These events are seared into the parents' minds, turning the first year into an eternity.

Monotony speeds up the perception of time.[252] The same routine day after day plasters no new posters to the wall; the mind has nothing to grasp onto to distinguish one day from another (or one week or month from another). Time blends together and condenses down the amount of memory-space it occupies. A year of pure routine is commuted to months or weeks.

To recap, monotonous periods condense down in the mind (speeding time up), and novel experiences flare out (slowing time down). This altered time perception creates a time warp. Test it: do three new things in a day, and follow it with five days of pure routine. Looking back, that one day will seem longer than a day, expanded or slowed time, while the five hum-drum days will feel to have condensed down, or sped up. The feel of time, its nuance, depends on how many signposts are staked into the cortex of the brain.

Hyper-concentration has the same effect as monotony, slowing time. Imagine putting a jigsaw puzzle together; you're doing one continuous thing, so few signposts are erected, and hours can pass unnoticed. This state is referred to as *flow*, and can be helpful for pain patients because it's the ultimate distraction (a near out-of-body experience).

This concept of mental signposts and flow states has a paradoxical effect on the chronic pain patient. You'd expect pain to cause monotony, with a feeling of weeks and months flying by. But the opposite is true. Pain evolved to warn us of danger; there is nothing better to wrench the concentration away to focus on the hurt; this is how as cavemen, we escaped the biting tiger and survived. Pain creates an anti-flow state: an inability to concentrate on anything but the pain. Every twinge is a mini-sign post, searing into our brain a brand we can look back at. I recall all my $^{10}/_{10}$ pain days, because no matter how long we endure pain, we don't get used to it—pain remains a novelty, creating signposts, slowing time.

When pain is at its worst, sand stops slipping through the hourglass. We stop looking to the future, because what future can we envisage but one of pain? Short-term plans are chucked first: I won't be able to attend my son's music recital next month; then medium-term plans are tossed: I can't be a law student with such pain; and finally, the long-term plans are ditched: no one will want to marry me with chronic pain. Time at a stand-still, and the non-existence of future time, leads to a feeling of depersonalization,[253] loss of identity and a schizoid personality. A twilight zone.

Einstein used thought experiments to describe his complex theories; many dealt with the passage of time under different circumstances. One involves an observer on a speeding train heading towards a tree in the distance. A second observer is stationary on a platform, also looking towards the tree. A bolt of lightning strikes the tree as the two men line up in space, but with one stationary and the other at high velocity. The man on the speeding train observes the lightning strike before the man on the platform (as he is speeding towards the light that is in turn speeding towards him). If each man clicks a stopwatch when he sees the lightning strike, the clocks will differ. But whose clock is correct?

The answer is they are both correct, even though the two clocks show different times. The lightning only struck the tree one time, but each observer had a different "frame of reference," and within their respective frames of reference they are both correct in when they see the lightning strike. (Einstein won a Nobel prize for these thought experiments, so don't worry if it boggles your mind).

When a pain patient sees her doctor, she and the doctor have different frames of reference, observing the movement of time at different speeds. The doctor is busy, hyper-concentrated and in a state of "flow," and so time for him is condensed down (sped-up). The patient is in pain, hammering signposts in throughout her day, causing time dilation (a slowing down). If she starts a medication that requires "awhile" to see an effect, she will return after two weeks (which felt like 2 months), saying she's been on the drug long enough to know its not working. The doctor, observing from the platform with a different stop watch, is in a different frame of reference, and may not appreciate his patient's time warp. This muddles the adage "tincture of time"— because a tincture of whose time?

Einstein's space-time continuum dealt with the fourth dimension and actual changes in time in relation to the speed of light. My pain-time continuum deals with the perception of time, and how events can snarl how long things "seem." We are in a time warp compared to the rest of the world, which is eerie and leads to existential thinking. A good pain doctor will understand his patients are disconnected from reality (calming the frantic patient who saw lightning strike a tree, explaining it hasn't happened yet, but will soon).

The final quirk of pain and time to note is pain's incrementalism. Pain improves or worsens so slowly as to be imperceptible to the patient. A 1% change every month will feel like no change over a half year (6%). But if the patient keeps a pain journal, and looks back two years later, she'll recognize the pain has improved 24%, which is not an insignificant amount. Recognizing this will make her feel better, even though her pain feels the same as six months ago. A pain journal anchors you to real world "time," preventing getting sucked up into the pain-time continuum.

Enough is enough.

You Find Out Who Your Friends Are

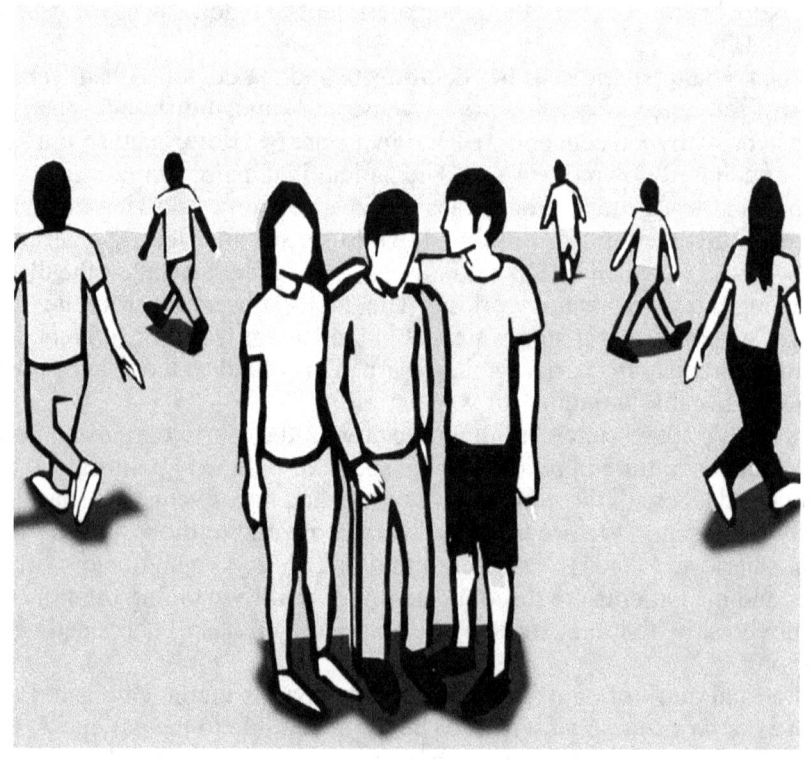

"A silver lining in the dark cloud of serious illness—your own or a loved one's—is the help and caring offered by friends, and the way that help can deepen friendships."

—*New York Times*, Deborah Tannen[254]

For many years after the onset of my pain, I purposely moved and lived far from my parents. My agony was ruining their lives; so I figured I'd go off by myself, as dogs do to die, and just suffer. But this was hiding from my problems, or hiding my problems from others. I could pretend on the phone I was doing fine, but I couldn't pretend when they were present in the same room as me.

Part of the shock of incurable pain is the instability of friendships. We take friendships for granted; they come and go as we move between cities, switch jobs and enter and leave relationships. I didn't give it a second thought, assuming I could always make new friends. But extend friends to include an entire social network of family, partners, colleagues, acquaintances and even strangers. Each adds value to your life in ways you don't realize.

> The message that emerges loud and clear from scientific evidence accumulated since the mid-1970s is that having a reasonable quantity and quality of social relationships is essential for mental and physical well-being. Loneliness and social isolation can inflict greater damage on our health than social stress.[255]

Pain patients cling to friends like a buoy in a choppy sea, but this sudden dependence is unwelcome. As the emotional and physical needs increase, your friends will feel the tug of obligation as you parasitize their schedules and orderly lives. Emotions are contagious, and the fear emanating from you will be draining. Eventually the veil will lift and the façade will crumble and many will reveal themselves as fair-weather friends. They will cut off the diseased appendage restricting their lives—you. This is how I felt when I was on the wrong end of the amputation, again and again.

As the weather turns stormy, each friend will turn their cards and reveal their hand—their boundary. This is their commitment point beyond which they will not pass: some will drive you to appointments, but not wait during the procedure. Others will allow you to stay in their extra room, but not take a day off work to be with you. Some will drop off food and flowers at your door, but not physically show their presence in your life. And for most there is no line of involvement, they will fade from your life permanently.

But angels exist, who have with no boundary line of involvement. Treasure them. They will disrupt their lives to assist in your care, and you'll be surprised how a distant relative or mere acquaintance will step up to the plate, while a "best friend" disappears. It's a matter of selflessness, which is totally unpredictable. In any case, knowing an angel benefits you in many ways other than the actual physical help. They can modulate your stress by being present, promoting healthier behavior: "Social isolation can foster self-destructiveness: it's all too easy to give in to temptation and indulge in that extra ice cream, cigarette or glass or whiskey. The presence of friends or relations on the other hand tends to modulate our potential excesses for fear of incurring social disapproval."[256] Friends can tell when you're not quite right, help financially with emergency loans and their detachment allows an objectivity for the many decisions to make. A second set of eyes at a busy intersection.

Making Friends

How do you make new friends with chronic pain? To form social connections you must first have social interactions, and to have social interactions you must leave the house and…interact. Whether it is a pain support group, a book club, a PTA meeting or the monthly neighborhood watch meeting, Dale Carnegie's advice is useful: "You can make more friends in two months by becoming interested in other people than you can in two years by trying to get people interested in you."

You've lost friendships since the pain began, so don't make the same mistakes again; when you meet new people don't allow pain to become the focal point of conversation. Mention it in passing, and then become truly interested in the new people you meet. I get a mood lift from interacting with the people I pay to provide services: my massage therapist, psychologist, physician, house cleaner and even the people I see in coffee shops and restaurants I visit. Join clubs, a gym, take a class or go to www.meetup.com and browse for others seeking social interaction. Do you know the neighbors living on your street or in your building? Knock on doors and invite them over. Join a Toastmasters club.

Once you've met someone, you need to cultivate the friendship. The biggest impediment to this is pain's unreliability, which leads to last minute cancelations. Begin slowly, and start with things you know you'll be less likely to cancel. My two foolproof rules to making friends are: 1) ask people about themselves and 2) remember their names.

Surgery

After my first surgery one complication snowballed into another: pneumonia, opioid withdrawal and the inability to urinate requiring discharge with a urinary catheter in place. The demand on my friends grew and their varying levels of availability became apparent. A recent person I'd been dating didn't visit for my entire ten-day hospitalization, yet an associate from work came every day. I hardly knew her, yet she helped me dress, get to the bathroom and checked on my progress. She was an angel.

I was angry at my friends' lack of involvement, abandoning me in a time of need. In retrospect I realize people are different, and you can't change them into what you want them to be. Don't cut off friends for these human shortcomings, because your circle of friends will naturally constrict as your disease progresses. Forgive behavior you would normally not tolerate; swallow your pride. Take from each what they are willing to give for as long as they are willing to, give it the morale of this chapter.

When I was a medical student I remember being at a fellow student's house during a party and finding pinned to his cork-board the following list.

Age 26: Graduate medical school.
Age 30: Graduate residency.
Age 32-35: Get married.
Age 35: Buy house.
Age 35–40: Have children.

I passed the list around the party and we all had a laugh at his expense. But I've often thought back to that pithy list. He wrote down what we all mentally outline. We have goals and time frames mapped out, even if we don't enumerate them as he did.

Chronic pain tears the neatly organized list into a million little pieces. The key is being able to find all those bits of paper, rearrange them, tape them back together, and still be able to read the list. Chronic pain will cause some scraps to fly out the window and go missing forever. Some bits you will find, but won't fit back into the jigsaw as smoothly as you'd like. The Scotch tape will run out and you may not be able to read your own handwriting. Putting the puzzle of life back together is difficult, but what is our alternative?

Ironically, my list resembled the one I once mocked. But as I picked up the bits of paper from the floor, wondering for the first time what had been written there, pieces seemed to be missing.

Age 30+: Work as a physician. (Missing!)
Age 32–35: Get married. (Gone!)
Age 40: Have children. (Has anyone seen that bit? I can't seem to find it.)

I decided to start a new list from scratch. I decided to retrain in a different specialty, to be a pain doctor (fitting, no?). I filled out the applications, got letters of recommendation, and was invited for a few interviews. I interviewed at Stanford first: After a long discussion with the chairman we both agreed I wasn't strong enough to stand wearing the lead aprons needed for radiation shielding. Darn, another smudge on my list. And on it went.

My advice is to keep writing the list. It'll be frustrating to see things written scratched off immediately. But keep going. Job B doesn't work? Try Job C, or D. Be nimble and adjust as your pain waxes and wanes, but realistic in what jobs you can physically perform.

Goals

After my first two years of pain, all I wanted was to walk around the block without pain; a reasonable goal for someone who formally ran every day and was a varsity tennis captain in high school. Gradually my pain lessened and I was able to walk around the block. Goal achieved. Small goals improve everyday living and ward off all the secondary diagnoses that make up chronic pain syndrome.

By keeping your ambition in check and not getting greedy, you can enjoy the best of your goal's benefits and none of the dangers of overreaching. Patients with pain need goals as much as they need food and water. Goals help you get out of bed in the morning, shower, and dress. They prompt you to mail a package at the post office, or invite friends for dinner.

When you hurt, you avoid doing the day-to-day things that cause you pain. Doing anything is a chore. Yet bear in mind the quick, three-step decline into total isolation and self-neglect that results from inaction. First, you withdraw from social interactions. You stop returning phone calls and become a hermit. Secondly, you ignore your housework: You stop cleaning, the dishes stack up with the garbage, bills go unpaid, and laundry piles up. You finally stop caring for yourself. You stop eating, don't shower, or even get out of bed. This cycle leads to severe depression and physical deconditioning, which loops back and worsens your pain.

Avoid this spiral by setting small goals for yourself on a weekly schedule. Monday, get groceries, and save Tuesday for the post office. Dry cleaning is for Wednesday, and return the library books Thursday. With time, you will find the right balance between the errands and your ability to be active each day. If you overbook, you'll end up in pain. If you under-book a week, you'll fall behind in your daily activities. These small, frequent goals will add structure to your life and get you out of the house. Checking things off a written checklist also provides satisfaction and a feeling of purpose, and increases your physical activity.

Take from each what they are willing to give.

The Disability Treadmill

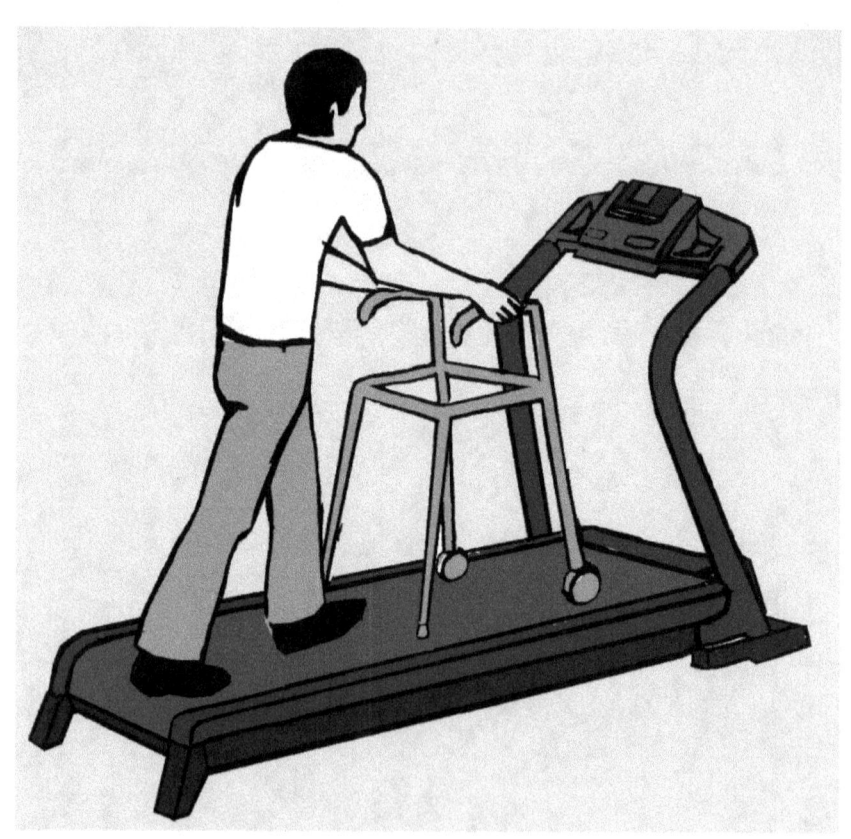

"Dogs bark, but the caravan moves on."

—Arabic Proverb

With chronic pain, you will get used to being different. But society isn't familiar yet with all the paraphernalia that a pain patient has to stitch together to get through a day. I use a sock donner to put my socks on, and all my furniture has risers to increase the sitting height. I use a firm chair insert for my car and can never ride in a car with poor shock absorbers. I have my special cushion for movie theater seats, and a pick-up stick to grab things up off the ground. I replaced my refrigerator so the fridge is on top and freezer on the bottom so I no longer have to bend to get food. I have ice packs ready to go and a cooler to transport them. I have hot packs for my toes and a cart to move my laundry. I pay Safeway to deliver my groceries and an assistant for weekly tasks. I hire a dog walker for the flare-up days. I wear a back brace I fashioned myself, and strategically follow people through heavy doors at the mall, avoiding having to open them myself. I call ahead to restaurants to reserve a table with a hard-backed chair. I only take elevators, and feel lost without my handicapped placard. I ask for help. I ask for help. I ask for help.

Strangers seem to derive satisfaction from helping me lift and move things. The requests I make brightens their mood, especially doing their good deed for the day in front of friends. Don't be timid about asking anyone for help. Each of these workarounds helps a little; and I make it by. Here I am finishing a book after ten years of pain. And always, medical science advances.

To Work or Not to Work

In our society our identity is connected to our jobs, and we are even introduced by our job titles, such as "Bill the lawyer." When we stop working and become non-contributors to society, we lose part of our identity. In the movie *About a Boy*, Hugh Grant suffers the dilemma of how to answer the question, "What do you do for a living?" His response: "I don't...actually, do anything." Stone cold silence is what he gets back in return, as do I when I answer similarly. The answer sends people jumping to their own conclusions about why you don't work, that you have a trust fund or are lazy. Is a better answer a fifteen-minute story about what you used to do, and how much pain you still have? The better answer is to return to work. Any work.

With this comes the consideration of disability, and a professional assessment of your ability to work. You will be scrutinized and the question will be asked why you are uniquely unable to work. Look at it from the clinician's perspective, with the unenviable task of objectively assessing a subjective quantity: pain.

The first disability question asked is are you able to do any job? The second question is if there's a job you are able to do, to what extent are you able to do it? How part-time do you need, and what accommodations need to be made for your disability? Psychosocial factors are a significant determinant in a person's ability to return to work, such as depression or other psychiatric illnesses resulting from the chronic pain, as well as the support system a patient has at home to aid their return to work. It is important, therefore, for Occupational Therapists and Social Workers to have an understanding of these factors when evaluating a person's ability to return to work.

Once we qualify as disabled, our society has few safety nets for people whose chronic medical conditions prevent them from working regular hours. They are defined below in increasing order of value they provide to the recipient.

- Supplemental Security Income (SSI): Federal insurance for those who haven't worked or who have not worked enough to qualify for SSDI. These recipients receive Medicaid as well as a small monthly stipend.
- Social Security Disability (SSDI): Federal insurance for those who have accumulated enough work credits to qualify. This group receives Medicare and a larger monthly stipend.
- Employer-supplied disability policies: This includes worker's compensation as well as work provided disability policies (which many people are not aware they even have until they need it).
- Private disability policies: Private policies are bought with after-tax dollars, thus, their payouts are 100 percent tax-free. Many times these policies are job-specific.

SSI and SSDI are piecemeal federal policies meant to supplement employer supplied or private disability policies. But there is an elephant in the room; once receiving payments from one or more of these disability policies, many patients remain on them indefinitely. They remain on the disability treadmill. Even with improvement in health, many patients still elect to remain on disability. What prevents them from removing themselves from their disability programs is not laziness or incapacity, but fear. This is a particular problem for pain patients because of the propensity for pain flare-ups. We fear returning to work and then finding ourselves unable to perform because of pain. This is rational, but not the best choice for many reasons.

These safety nets all have programs to give patients with chronic disease incentive to return to work. Many have long trial periods where you can return to the comfort of being on disability without having to reapply. Most let you keep your health insurance and even allow you to work part-time, ad infinitum.

With SSI, you are able to work until your earnings exceed your SSI payments. If this happens and you at some point become sick again, you have five years during which time you can jump right back onto SSI without having to reapply. Five years. In addition, you are able to deduct work-related expenses from your income to lower your income as much as possible: transportation costs, retraining costs, tuition, etc. You even get to keep your Medicaid. The policy is straightforward: "After you return to work, your Medicaid coverage can continue, even if your earnings (alone or in combination with your other income) become too high for an SSI cash payment."[257]

SSDI has a more formalized "Ticket to Work" program, which provides free training and vocational services. You have a six-month trial work period. If during this period you earn less than $720 per month, nothing will be affected. If you earn more you have a "trial work period" for nine months followed by an "extended period of eligibility" which lasts for three and a half years. You keep your Medicare benefits for eight and a half years, even after SSDI payments stopped.

Employer-provided policies, workers compensation and private disability policies all have incentives to allow you to return to work. My policies have a graduated decrease in payments depending on how much I earn: for every dollar I earn, the policy will pay me 25 cents less. If I earn over a certain amount the ratio changes until I am back to earning my full salary. And if you are approved for SSI or SSDI and owe government backed student loans, there is a process by which these loans can be totally discharged (go to www.disabilitydischarge.com).

These programs want you to return to work, and understand the trepidation sick people have giving up hard-fought benefits. The average waiting period for SSDI is three years. Many of these incentive-based programs are salary-based, too; and remember, you decide what your salary is going to be by how much you work. If you can only work part-time, then do that, and continue to collect partial disability payments beyond your part-time salary. This is not taking advantage of the system, but it is how the system is supposed to work.

No one reading this book is as disabled as Stephen Hawking, the famous physicist who has a progressive motor neuron disease called ALS. Yet he travels, writes books, and continues to do his research in theoretical physics even though his condition has deteriorated to the point where he can now only raise one eyebrow. When you think you are too sick to be able to return to work, go to Stephen Hawking's website and read the section he writes on how he deals with his disability.[258] It will inspire you to stick your toe back into the job market.

When you return to work you will reestablish your identity and your social worth to society. You will become less isolated as you are forced to socialize with coworkers. You'll have a schedule and routine, grounding you.

You will gain a sense of satisfaction and your skills will stop eroding. Your value to society, your sense of community, and your earnings will all increase. Work will distract you from your pain, and return to you an identity—a title. Work returns to you much of what chronic pain steals.

Jumping off the Treadmill

My return to work began with the writing of this book. At the time it was all I was able to do, after two back surgeries in succession totally incapacitated me. With time, my pain didn't improve, but my coping abilities did. I ventured out and started interviewing for jobs. I looked for teaching jobs, medical expert jobs, chart review jobs, and consultant jobs. Some failed to pan out. The rest were unable to accommodate my disability requirements, so I decided to try and return to medicine in a different specialty.

Failing those attempts I decided to go into business for myself. I saved my disability checks for 2 years, and started buying foreclosed homes at auctions, fixing them up with the help of workers I found, and renting them out. I managed to buy one a year over the last few years. I now have a nice stream of positive income. Part of my objective was to get enough positive cash flow to survive if my disability policies decided to stop paying or went bankrupt, as almost happened during the financial collapse. These few houses gave me a sense of security, prompting me to look at riskier jobs (from a disability standpoint).

Even your humble author is not immune from the fear of jumping off of the disability treadmill. What gives you the sense of security you need to take the plunge back to work? Hire a lawyer to review your disability contracts and tell you what will happen if you return to work. Or start a small business, maybe selling products on eBay, until you have enough financial security to become employed as you were before. Or work a job that pays cash. It has taken me ten years to get to this point, so I do not judge anyone else's incrementalism in returning to work. No matter how slow you move, move. Take steps, fail, and take more steps. The benefits you get from work are many; the risks less than you probably think.

Return To Work.

Dark Night of the Soul

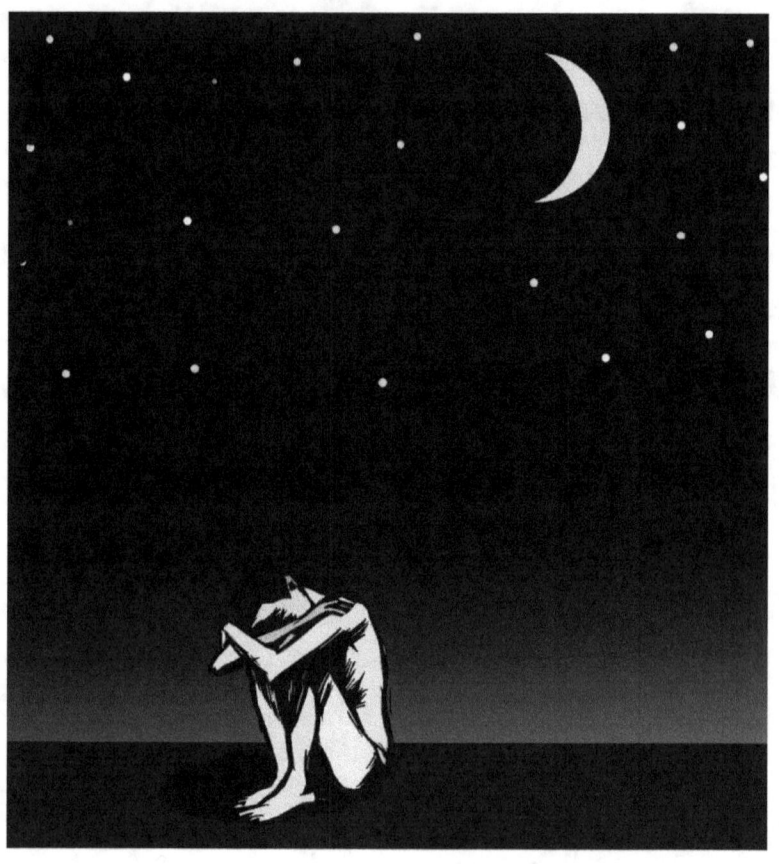

"I can't go on. I'll go on."

—Samuel Beckett

Awareness that pain will last forever, and abandoning treatments to cure or improve pain, is not acceptance of pain. Those first two steps are easy to see—billboard signs along a freeway—but are less than halfway to journey's end. The next turn off is not as obvious. I erect the signpost Dark Night of the Soul, but call it what you want—it's off-road and unmapped.

To accept pain, you must incorporate it into your being. And to do so requires a dismantling of your identity, selfhood and ego. A clearing out of the old to allow room for the new. Destruction, followed by rebuilding. Disintegration, followed by reintegration. Deprogramming, followed by reprogramming.

Books on pain avoid this chapter because it doesn't help sell books. But it's a reality. You enter a dark night with a longing for your old self and the way things used to be. But as the months turn into years, yearning turns into mourning, accompanied by depression, hopelessness and loneliness. You're in purgatory, and nothing will curtail this process but to push forward and emerge from the other side. While painful, it's a positive experience, because after this deworlding the reworlding can begin.[259]

The Universality of the Dark Night

The phrase Dark Night of the Soul was first coined as a spiritual crisis when Christians lost belief in God. But it's transgressed religion and become a metaphor for any period of transformation in life. Some will have repetitive dark nights, while others one extended darkness. Many will deny the experience, and others will fail to recognize it, allowing it to pass unrequited. It can be internally driven, a period of depression, or externally imposed with a prison sentence, illness or car accident.

The theme is present in many religious offshoots: Kabbalah within Judaism, Sufism within Islam, Vedanta within Hinduism and Gnosticism within Christianity. Buddhists travel through the knowledge of suffering (dark night) to attain enlightenment (the rebuilding). The Hindus seek moksh, and the Christians have the crucified Christ—"My God, my God, why have you forsaken me?"—who then rises to heaven.

Mythology represents it by imprisonment, crucifixion, dismemberment and abduction: "experiences traditionally weathered by sun-gods and heroes: Gilgamesh, Osiris, Christ, Dante, Odysseus, Aeneas."[260] Jonah is swallowed into the belly of a whale, and Zen Buddhists descend "into the cave of the blue dragon."[261]

Psychology also acknowledges the experience, with Jung referring to it as a night sea journey. There is a "descent into Hades and a journey to the land of ghosts somewhere beyond this world, beyond consciousness, hence an immersion in the unconscious."[262] The dark night is a questioning of existence necessary to arrive at a higher spiritual plane, broadening of consciousness or deeper awareness of oneself.

Famous Dark Nights

Astronomist Galileo Galilei was put under house arrest for claiming the Earth revolved around the Sun. During this time he wrote his finest work, *Two New Sciences*. Sir Thomas More, advisor to King Henry VIII, refused to acknowledge his divorce and title as head of the Church of England. He was convicted of treason and beheaded, but his correspondences from prison are also his most famous writings.

Playwright Oscar Wilde, imprisoned for homosexuality, transitioned from a life of opulence to one of "hard labour, hard fare and a hard bed." Isolated and with deteriorating health, he wrote his most famous work, *De Profundis*, during this time. His emergence led to spiritual growth and a promise never to forget the darkness: "My only mistake was that I confined myself so exclusively to the trees of what seemed to me the sun-lit side of the garden, and shunned the other side for its shadow and its gloom."[263]

Nelson Mandela was imprisoned for twenty-seven years on Robben Island; during this time he became the most famous person in Africa from his prison correspondence, and was elected president in 1994. Mother Teresa described her dark night in letters posthumously released, "[T]he silence and the emptiness is so great, that I look and do not see,—Listen and do not hear … [there is a] terrible pain of loss, of God not wanting me, of God not being God, of God not really existing."

Writer Eckhart Tolle describes a "collapse of … the meaning that you had given your life, your activities, your achievements, where you are going, what is considered important."[264] After passing through his night, he further reflects, "I woke up and everything was so peaceful. The peace was there because there was no self. Just a sense of presence or 'beingness.'"[265]

The Flotsam and Jetsam of your Old Self

To effect radical transformation a dark night must be harsh and punishing to destroy the embedded self and instinctual ways of doing things. To retrain muscle memory in the new motions of tomorrow there must first be an annihilation of the ego—the land between the conscious and unconscious. The "who you are" is destroyed, which is so ingrained it's analogous to tearing down a skyscraper and clearing away the crumpled steel and debris—no easy task. Likewise, from wrecking ball to ribbon cutting, your dark night will seem endless.

Our night is imposed by an external illness causing internal pain. It will carry on well after our breaking point; it must, because if it ends too soon we'll think we can turn around and regain our old life. We must snap, and remain in darkness beyond this point, to know we can't regress. And danger exists during this time, for we will all contemplate suicide as a quick exit.

During my dark night I was directionless—a boat adrift at sea. Half the time I directed my own medical care, the other half I moved without a rudder through hospitals and clinics, pharmacies and therapists. I felt so alone on my night sea journey I pushed my remaining friends away, and turned to alcohol to keep myself afloat. But this only blurred the compass, keeping me at sea longer.

A boat in peril jettisons its cargo overboard to lighten its load—the floating cargo is called jetsam. I shed the jetsam of my former, pain-free self—playing sports, hiking, biking, having a large social circle and performing a full day's work—to unencumber myself and speed my way through the darkness. But there is only so much cargo to heave overboard; the rest is structure, the boat itself.

When a ship crashes against the rocks, the breakage of the boat is called flotsam. When I crashed, my ego and selfhood broke into a million pieces of flotsam as I arrived at midnight. But halfway to dawn is still halfway back to dusk. The night continued until the early hours of the morning, when pinholes of light broke through the canopy of blackness. A new friend appeared and a new physician signed on. I followed the pinholes, putting myself back together. The months and years continued to pass and larger stars twinkled—I was accepted for Social Security Disability and found Janelle, my physical therapist. But the dark night didn't end when it should have, because deep vestiges of my old self still needed uprooting. I waited, and more stars appeared—a new apartment, a new medication. Only when I'd given up on ever escaping did a north star appear—and a new surgeon— guiding me as it has so many travelers over the centuries.

Only when it's truly dark can you see the stars.

Escaping the Rabbit Hole

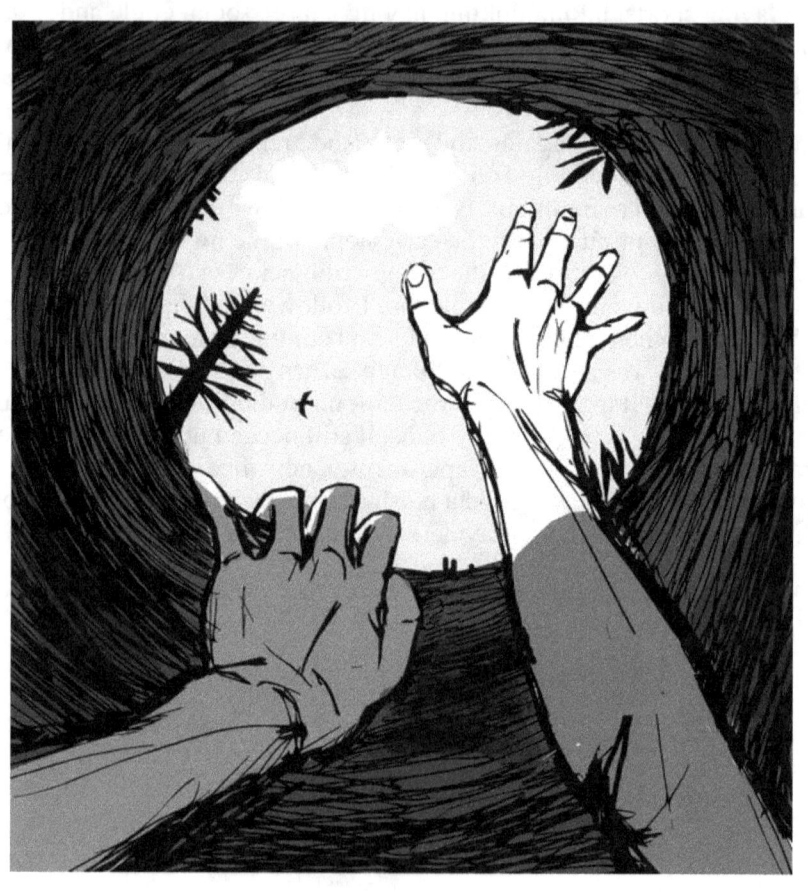

"To live is to suffer, to survive is to find meaning in the suffering. If there is a purpose in life at all, there must be a purpose in suffering and dying."

—Victor Frankl

Victor Frankl was a psychiatrist held captive at Auschwitz during the Holocaust, and his experience epitomizes a dark night of the soul. Broken down to a sack of rags and flesh, in the midst of a genocide with prisoners dying around him,[266] he found a path out of the dark night and developed a coping mechanism allowing him and others to survive the cruel conditions. After the Holocaust, this enlightenment led to a new form of psychoanalysis called logotherapy—uncovering a person's purpose in life. His in-camp coping strategy, and logotherapy, are both applicable to chronic pain.

Frankl foresaw prisoners' deaths days beforehand because they exhibited the same symptom—a loss of future meaning.[267] They then progressed through a series of steps: refusing to get out of bed, converse and eat until they lay festering in their own excrement until death. A psychological loss of purpose led to a corporal physical decline.

This mind-body connection interested Frankl, because the prisoners seemed to will themselves to death. One prisoner had a dream of liberation so vivid it included a date and time. When that day came and went and "the expected liberation did not come … [it] suddenly lowered his body's resistance against the latent typhus infection. His faith in the future and his will to live had become paralyzed and his body fell victim to illness."[268]

Loss of purpose rapidly causing death led Frankl to consider the reverse: Can creating meaning, a future goal, instill a will to live? Would mental purpose strengthen the physical body? He began therapy with his fellow prisoners, reminding them life still expected something from them. One prisoner had a child he wanted to return to, and another a manuscript yet to be published. He reinforced the importance of these goals, which strengthened their coping skills and led both men to survive. "A man who becomes conscious of the responsibility he bears towards a human being who affectionately waits for him, or to an unfinished work, will never be able to throw away his life."[269]

Frankl reminded prisoners why they were holding onto life, linking their pain to a future purpose. A single-mindedness then overcame them, and their wretched conditions became more tolerable.[270] There is no true comparison of the external suffering of these death camps, but the coping mechanism of attaching meaning to pain can be applied to our internal suffering.

The Meaning of Life

Nietzsche proposed humans have a will to power: to dominate and expand their authority and wealth. This was followed by Freud's will to pleasure, where sexual gratification is the primary motivating force. Frankl's logotherapy—the Third Viennese School of Psychotherapy—is a will to meaning. Each person has a purpose to fulfill, and life's meaning is the discovery and pursuit of this purpose.[271]

> [L]ife holds a potential meaning under any conditions, even the most miserable ones. And I thought that if the point were demonstrated in a situation as extreme as that in a concentration camp ... it might be helpful to people who are prone to despair.[272]

After the Holocaust Frankl sought to unmask purpose in his patient's lives. They'd present with a myriad of problems, which he'd bypass and ask, "What's keeping you from simply killing yourself?" The answer to this question was the meaning of their life—their will to live.

One patient was distressed because his wife had died, and he didn't know how to continue without her. Frankl asked the man what if it had been he who had died, and his wife who had lived. He answered she would have suffered terribly without him to support her. Pointing out he was enduring this suffering in his wife's stead, Frankl ascribed meaning to this man's grief. He could now revel in his suffering, knowing each pang of mourning was pain his wife would not feel.

The Meaning of Pain

Living a life without meaning is living in an existential vacuum, with the remaining days measured out in web-clicks. Chronic pain makes it easy to slip into this vacuum; we personify the sick role, illness behavior and are exempt from duties and engagements. We pity ourselves, take pills that zonk us out as the disability treadmill whirrs. What meaning is there to such a life?

Well, answer Frankl's intake question: What's keeping you from killing yourself? I still ask myself this question because my answer changes (along with my life's meaning). Working as a physician gave my life purpose and fulfillment; but that disappeared and I got stuck for years lying on my mother's couch—my cot—while the invisible beatings tore at me daily. There was no fear of imminent death, but the internal fear of being in pain forever.

I started small, looking for day-to-day meaning to my pain. One day I fell in agony as I bent to unload clothes from the dryer. As I sat on the floor, clothes everywhere, I felt humbled. This is not an adjective ever used to describe doctors. But why? I became determined to bring that humility back to the hospital with me, to not be the rushed doctor who doesn't makes eye contact. A moment of pain gave me insight still with me today.

I looked past my pain to the add-on diagnosis of Chronic Pain Syndrome I've collected: anxiety, depression, alcoholism and social withdrawal. I can feel the addict's craving, the nellie's butterflies, the wretch's glumness and the hermit's avoidance. This is my current residency, which will better qualify me to treat these diagnoses when or if I do return to practice medicine.

You're holding today's purpose in your hands, this book. I wouldn't have written a book on pain, or any book, if I hadn't lived through this last decade. When pain leads to a problem, I solve it, and it becomes something to write about. As I utilize my pain, it recedes into the background as its purpose moves to the foreground, and more chapters emerge.

Emerging from the Rabbit Hole

Alice in Wonderland was pulled out of her rabbit hole when her sister woke her. Victor Frankl was presented with the same situation, but chose differently:

> I was roused one night by the groans of a fellow prisoner, who threw himself about in his sleep, obviously having a horrible nightmare. ... I drew back the hand which was ready to shake him ... no dream, no matter how horrible, could be as bad as the reality of the camp which surrounded us, and to which I was about to recall him.[273]

We've all fallen down a rabbit hole and won't be rousted anytime soon. We need to make sense of our altered world, give it meaning, and make it a wonderland. Frankl's survival and transformation gives me solace during hard times. He describes the sky black with the soot and ashes of the burning bodies of the crematorium, creating a literal dark night to accompany the figurative.

His midnight occurred when thoughts of suicide disappeared from his mind, because the remaining life was worth less than the effort to extinguish it. Broken down beyond his surrender point, his ego shattered and he became aware of the suffering around him. Terror was replaced by calm, and in the midst of hell Frankl was reborn into a higher state of consciousness. As the fires of the crematorium burned around him, he untied the ropes mooring other prisoners, setting them off on their own dark sea voyages.

Find meaning in your pain.

Pain Willingness

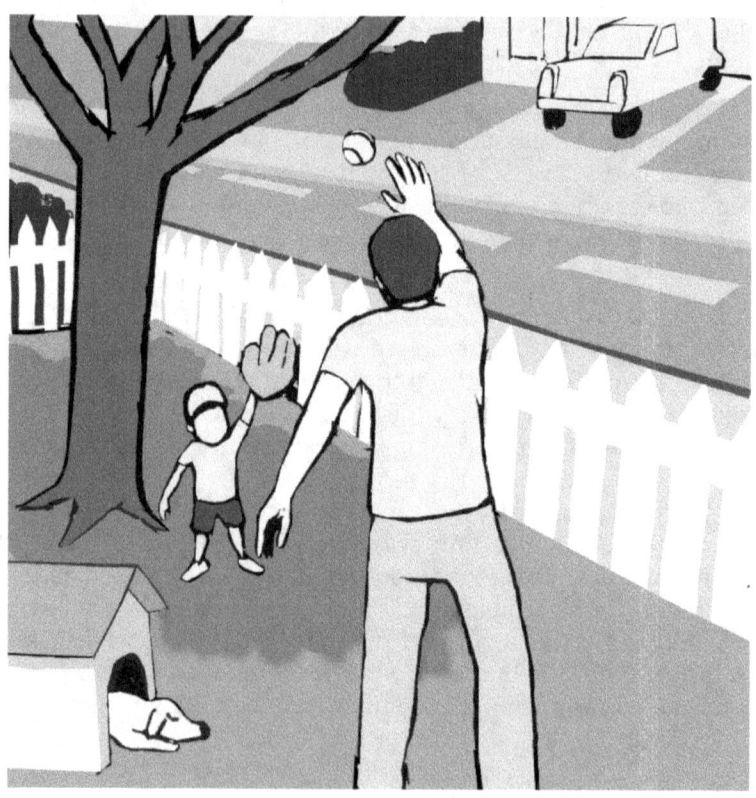

"And those who were seen dancing were thought to be insane by those who could not hear the music."

—Fredrich Nietzsche

Chronic pain, most of the time, is chronic.

Accept this, and evidence shows you'll know less pain intensity, anxiety, depression, isolation, disability and medication use. This finding doesn't correlate with pain severity, but with the degree of pain acceptance.[274] It's counter-intuitive: partaking in painful activities lessens pain. I explain it this way. Pain has an emotional component, which responds to antidepressants, and a pathologic component, best treated with pain killers. All pain is a combination of the two, emotional pain and pathologic pain.

Cherished physical activities exacerbate pathological pain and ease emotional pain; the sum of the two results in a payoff, a net decrease in pain—it's worth your while. The inverse, pain avoidance, robs life of precious moments; worsening emotional pain more than the "taking it easy" diminishes pathologic pain, resulting in a debt—a net worsening of pain. Exertion brings both gain and loss; but seven studies, across four countries, prove the gain outweighs the loss. [275]

Pain Willingness versus Pain Avoidance

Pain acceptance is referred to as pain willingness in the medical literature. It's defined as:[276]

- Acknowledging you have chronic pain.
- Experiencing pain without disturbing thoughts or anxiety.
- Committing yourself to move towards things valued in life.
- Responding to pain without attempts at control or avoidance.
- Abandoning unproductive efforts to control or cure your pain.
- Abandoning beliefs that pain impairs function, indicates harm or is disabling.

Pain avoidance is the inverse of each of these. This definition is like the curse of the Ten Commandments—impossible to obey (for who cannot covet?). I can't keep to the definition of pain acceptance, but I use it as a model to strive towards. A spectrum exists, with willingness and avoidance at each end, and we must edge towards the ideal of pain willingness. We must lean into the pain.[277]

Other Paths to Acceptance

I am a person with pain, not a person in pain. My old self is gone, and a new is self is reborn with pain intertwined. This Phoenix Model—identity destruction followed by a rising from the ashes—may not be your path to acceptance. Here are other paths from surveys of chronic pain patients.

- Control—control pain and don't give in to it.
- Day to day—accept a life of uncertainty, live in the present.
- Modification—change life to fit within the limits imposed by pain.
- Selectivity—avoid aspects of life that pain impacts, focus on pleasure.
- Loss of self—create a new identity incorporating pain (my path).
- No loss of self—don't let pain change who you are; focus life away from pain.
- Go with the flow—pain just happens; don't fight unwinnable battles.
- Spiritual—reach acceptance through spirituality.[278]

I've used the others, such as go with the flow, modification and selectivity; and when my pain was at its worst, I lived day-to-day. Whichever you choose, they all reach to the same goal—acceptance.

My Path

My trail had four switchbacks:

- Awareness—I realized the pain would be present forever.
- Abandonment—I ended the search for a cure and further treatment.
- Annihilation—My old self was destroyed.
- Acceptance—I created a new identity with pain.

Awareness is recognizing pain won't go away, and is terrifying. I conceded this quickly, because I've observed untreatable diseases, and know medicine's limits. I was getting my blood drawn one day, when the concept of incurability hit me. (The only other time I felt such terror was when I was ten years old, and I became aware that I was alive, and would die someday.)

Abandonment came slower. Bewilderment replaced terror, as I moved from treatment to treatment, and medication to medication. The doctors pushed, and inertia did the rest. I knew my pain was incurable, but not...untreatable. Putting a foot down—abandoning cure—slowed my movement, but it took another two years to drop the second foot— abandoning treatment—and stop all motion. The doctors wouldn't propel me any further; I fired them all, and canceled everything.

Annihilation of the old me was also a trial. My pain was incurable and untreatable—but wasn't I the same person, with the same experiences? I clung to my old self—care-free, social, hard-working—refusing to admit the loss. But a loss needs to be mourned, so I grieved, and this hospice period lasted five years: my Dark Night of the Soul.

Acceptance arrived when the new strand—pain—interwove itself into a new braid. I knew it was finished one day when I pulled into a parking garage to see a movie with a new friend. I got out of the car, popped the trunk and grabbed my tempurpedic-steel seat insert. "What's that?" my friend asked.

"Oh, I have chronic pain and can't handle the theater seats," rolled off my tongue matter-of-factly. I didn't try to hide or explain it away; muscle memory grabbed the seat, now routine.

"Oh, okay." And that was that. New life with pain throughout— acceptance.

My New Identity

I can't run. I can't jump. I struggle to unload groceries from the car. I hobble up stairs and avoid steep hills. But I no longer walk with a cane, coop myself up or avoid painful activities. The ease with which I tell people "I have chronic pain" and transition to another topic is disarming. People equate chronic pain to I-have-a-brain-tumor, but I disclose it with a I-got-a-latte-yesterday effortlessness. The tradeoff of doing things, pain willingness, outweighs the sacrifice that follows.

I have greater depth and complexity: friendships valued before no longer satisfy, and activities enjoyed before the pain are now untenable. So I make new friends and pursue different hobbies. My vacations are dictated by my new identity, as is the car I drive, the job I will work and the relationships I will enter into. I approach this with excitement, not sadness for a life lost. So many live in the same house and work the same job their entire lives— chronic pain forces everything to change. Recall Frankl's logotherapy: find meaning to, or in, life.

Chronic pain caused a zig in my life when anesthesiology became undoable. I tried to zag back on track retraining as a pain management doctor, but this natural evolution was also beyond my capabilities. I bided my time and began writing this book. Then Fate braided me a new specialty: Addiction Medicine. This would bind together my knowledge of opioids and pain management, but without the back-breaking lead shielding or emergency procedures. This will be my second act; unless the sun sets on yet another Dark Night of the Soul, barring this noble calling.

Lean into the pain.

End-notes

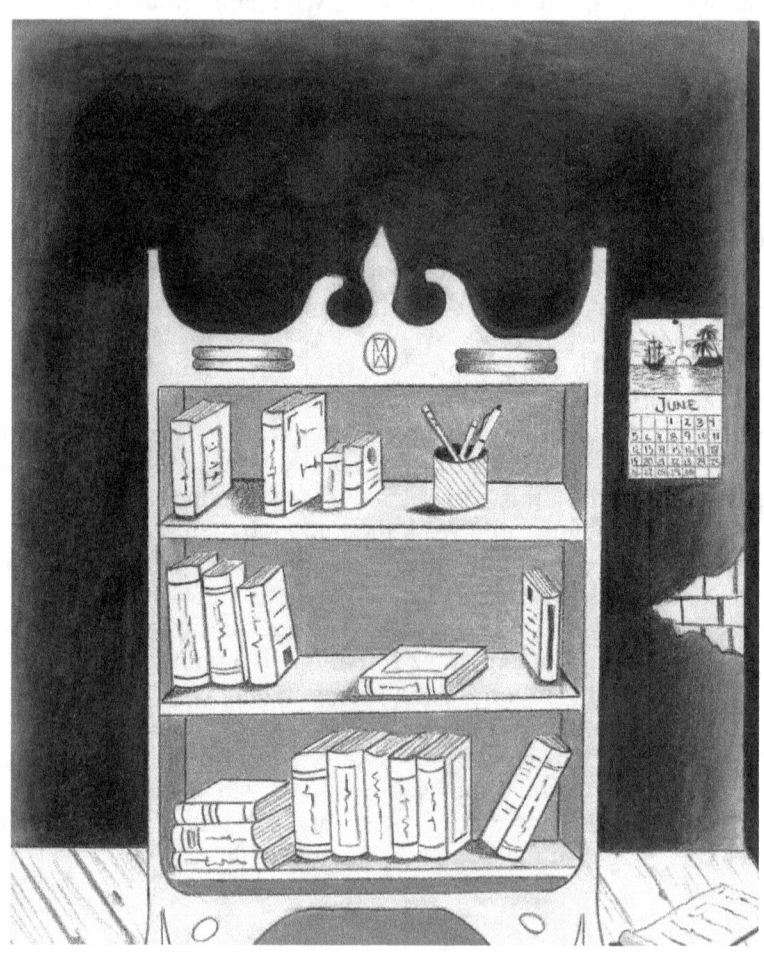

1 Institute of Medicine.

2 Hanson, *Coping with Chronic Pain*, 35.

3 A. L. Dewar, K. Gregg, M. I. White, J. Lander, "Navigating the health care system: perceptions of patients with chronic pain," Chronic Diseases in Canada, 29,4(2009):162-8.

4 Drew Pinsky M.D., http://transcripts.cnn.com/TRANSCRIPTS/1202/17/ddhln.01.html

5 Andrew Solomon, *The Noonday Demon* (New York, NY: Simon and Schuster 2001) 28.

6 Solomon, *Noonday Demon*, 71.

7 Flor, H., Turk, D., Birbaumer, N.,"Assessment of stress-related psychophysiological reactions in chronic back pain," Journal of Consulting and Clinical Psychology, 53,3 (1985):354-364.

8 Agüera, L., et al, "Medically unexplained pain complaints are associated with underlying unrecognized mood disorders in primary care," BMC Family Practice, 11(2010):17.

9 Ohayon MM. "Specific characteristics of the pain/depression association in the general population," J Clin Psychiatry. 2004;65(suppl12):5-9.

10 Ohayon MM, Schatzberg AF. "Using chronic pain to predict depressive morbidity in the general population," Arch Gen Psychiatry. 2003;60:39-47.

11 Wilson KG Mikail SF et al "Alternative diagnostic criteria for major depressive disorder in patients with chronic pain," Pain, (2001):227-234.

12 Hamilton, M. J. (1960). Neurology Neurosurgery and Psychiatry. Vol. 23: p. 56–62.

13 Lin, E., et al., "Effect of Improving Depression Care on Pain and Functional Outcomes Among Older Adults With Arthritis A Randomized Controlled Trial," JAMA, 290, 18(2003):2428-2429; Ahles TA, Wasson JH, Seville JL, et al. "A controlled trial of methods for managing pain in primary care patients with or without co-occurring psychosocial problems," Ann Fam Med. 2005;4:341-350.

14 Fishbain, D. Et al, "Chronic Pain-Associated Depression: Antecedent or Consequence of Chronic Pain? A Review," The Clinical Journal of Pain, 13,2(1997):116-137; Korff, M. Et al, "The Relationship Between Pain and Depression," The British Journal of Psychiatry, 168,30(1996):101-8.

15 http://www.nytimes.com/2012/01/25/health/depressions-criteria-may-be-changed-to-include-grieving.html?_r=1

16 60 Minutes, "Treating Depression," Feb. 19, 2012; http://www.cbsnews.com/8301-18560_162-57380893/treating-depression-is-there-a-placebo-effect/

17 Fournier, J., "Antidepressant Drug Effects and Depression Severity A Patient-Level Meta-analysis,"JAMA. 2010;303(1):47-53.

18 Rudy Severeijns et al., "Pain Catastrophizing Predicts Pain Intensity, Disability, and Psychological Distress Independent of the Level of Physical Impairment," 18(2001):165–172.

19 Luis F. Buenaver, Robert R. Edwards, Jennifer A. Haythornthwaite , "Pain-related Catastrophizing and Perceived Social Responses: Inter-relationships in the Context of Chronic Pain," Pain 127 (2007): 234-242.

20 Severeijns, "Pain Catastrophizing," 165-72.

21 Sullivan MJL, Bishop S, Pivik J., "The Pain Catastrophizing scale: development and validation," Psychol Assess 7 (1995): 524–32; Sullivan MJL, Neish N., "The effects of disclosure on pain during dental hygiene treatment: the moderating role of catastrophizing," Pain 79 (1999): 155–63.

22 Keefe FJ, et al., "Coping with rheumatoid arthritis: catastrophizing as a maladaptive strategy," Pain, 37(1989):51–6.

23 Bédard GB, et al., "Coping and self medication in a community sample of junior high school students," Pain Res Manage, 2(1997):151–6.

24 Robert R. Edwardsa, Michael T. Smitha, Ian Kudelb, Jennifer Haythornthwaite, "Pain-related catastrophizing as a risk factor for suicidal ideation in chronic pain," Pain, 15,126(2006):272-9.

25 Fordyce WE. "Behavioral methods for chronic pain and illness," Anesthesiology, 45,4(1976)471.

26 Gil KM, Abrams MR, Phillips G, et al. "Predicting health care use and activity level at 9-month follow-up," J Consult Clin Psychol, 60(1992):267–73.

27 Gil KM, et al."Sickle cell disease pain in children and adolescents: change in pain frequency and coping strategies over time," J Ped Psychol, 18(1993):621–637.

28 Michael J., et al., "Theoretical Perspectives on the Relation Between Catastrophizing and Pain," The Clinical Journal of Pain, 17(2001):52–64.

29 Turner JA, Clancy S., "Strategies for coping with chronic low back pain: relationships to pain and disability," Pain, 24(1986):355–64. Parker J.C., et al., "Pain control and rational thinking: implications for rheumatoid arthritis," Arthr Rheumatol, 32 (1989):984–90.; Keefe FJ, et al, "Pain coping skills training in the management of osteoarthritis knee pain: a comparative study," Behav Ther, 21(1991):49–62.

30 Prkachin, "Pain Behavior and the Development of Pain-Related Disability: The Importance of Guarding," Clin J Pain, 23,3(2007)270-277.

31 Prkachin, "Pain Behavior and the Development of Pain-Related Disability: The Importance of Guarding," Clin J Pain, 23,3(2007)270-277.

32 Fordyce WE. Behavioral methods for chronic pain and illness. (St. Louis: Mosby, 1976.)

33 Rhudy JL, Meagher MW. "Fear and anxiety: divergent effects on human pain thresholds," Pain 2000;84:65–75; Jorum E. "Noradrenergic mechanisms in mediation of stress- induced hyperalgesia in rats," Pain 1988;32:349–55.

34 Van Tulder, M.W., Assendelft, W.J.J., et al., "Spinal radiographic findings and non-specific low back pain," Spine,22(1997):427-434; Nachemson A Vingard E., "Assessment of patients with chronic pain: a best evidence synthesis," in Nachemson (ed) Neck and back pain: the scientific basis of causes, diagnosis and treatment (Philadelphia:Lippincott /Williams & Wilkins)189-235.

35 The New York Times, "Connecting the Neural Dots," 2/26/13.

36 Engel,"Psychogenic pain," 899-918.

37 See chapter "The Chronic Pain Syndrome."

38 Taddio, A.,"Effect of neonatal circumcision on pain response during subsequent routine vaccination," Lancet, 349 (1997):599-603.

39 Mazis, G., The trickster. magician and grieving man: Reconnecting men with earth. (Bear and Company, 1994); http://www.noharmm.org/zoske.htm;

Farrell, W., *The myth of male power: Why men are the disposable sex* (New York: Simon & Schuster, 1993); Goldberg, H., *The hazards of being male: Surviving the myth of masculine privilege* (New York: Signet Book,1976); Zoske, J., "Rethinking men's health and wellness," Wellness Management 12 (1996):1-6.

40 Engel GL: "Psychogenic pain and the pain prone patient," Am J Med 26 (1959): 899-918.

41 Severe and prolonged pain.
Pain in a pattern that doesn't correlate to the path of the nervous system.
No other pathological reason can be found for the pain.
The presence of psychological factors judged to be associated with the pain.
And one of the following three:
A temporal relationship between psychological conflict and pain exacerbation.
The pain enables the individual to avoid activity that is noxious to him or her.
The pain enables the patient to get support from the environment that might not otherwise be present.

42 Waddell G *The back pain Revolution* 2004 Churchill Livingston, Edinburgh; Hanson, *Coping with Chronic Pain*, 22.

43 Kelly Patrick Flannigan, MD, FRCP(C) "Pain is a blind guide in injury management" (1995).

44 Parsons, T., 7 Definitions of health and illness in the light of American values and social structure, (New York Free Press, 1958).

45 Maines, Rachel P., *The Technology of Orgasm: "Hysteria", the Vibrator, and Women's Sexual Satisfaction* (Baltimore: The Johns Hopkins University Press 1998).

46 Mechanic, D., Psychological Medicine, 1986, 16, 1-7, Gildenburg, P., *The chronic pain patient: Evaluation and management* (S Karger Pub: 1984)20.

47 "Persistent Pain as a Disease Entity: Implications for Clinical Management," Philip J. Siddall, Anesth Analg 2004;99:510 –20.

48 Miki K, Iwata K, Tsuboi Y, et al. "Dorsal column-thalamic pathway is involved in thalamic hyperexcitability following peripheral nerve injury: a lesion study in rats with experimen- tal mononeuropathy," Pain 2000;85:263–71; Gerke MB, Duggan AW, Xu L, Siddall PJ. "Thalamic neuronal activity in rats with mechanical allodynia following contusive spinal cord injury," Neuroscience 20003;117:715–22.

49 Ingvar M. "Pain and functional imaging," Phil Trans R Sc Lond 1999;354:1347–58; Chen AC. "New perspectives in EEG/MEG brain mapping and PET/fMRI neuroimaging of human pain," Int J Psychophysiol 2001;42:147–59; Treede RD, Kenshalo DR, Gracely RH, Jones AKP. "The cortical representation of pain," Pain 1999;79:105–11.

50 Jensen T Gottrup H Kasch H et al., "Has basic research contributed to chronic pain treatment?," Acta Anaes. Scand., 45, 9(2001):1128-1135; Curatolo M Petrersen-Felix S Arendt-Nielsen L et al., "Central hypersensitiivty in chronic pain after whiplash injury," Clinical Journal of Pain, 17,4(2001):306-315.

51 www.painco.co.uk/downloads/0412/041223/painmech-v3.doc

52 Dubner R., "Neural basis of persistent pain: sensory specialization, sensory modulation and neuronal plasticity," Progress in pain research and management, 8 (1997).

53 Descartes (1664).

54 http://www.sharkattacks.com/news1.htm

55 Skevington, Suzanne. *Psychology of pain* (New York: Wiley 1995)11.
56 Butler, *Explain Pain*, 8.
57 Beecher, H., "Relationship of significance of wound to pain experienced," JAMA, 161(1956):1604-1613.
58 Butler, *Explain Pain*, 16-21.
59 Smith, W.B., "The affects of experimenter gender on pain report in male and female subjects," Pain, 44(1991): 69-72.
60 Prkachin, "Pain Behavior and the Development of Pain-Related Disability: The Importance of Guarding," Clin J Pain, 23,3(2007)270-277.
61 Fordyce WE., *Behavioral methods for chronic pain and illness* (St Louis:Mosby 1976).
62 Lousberg R, Schmidt AJM, "The relationship between spouse solicitouness and pain behavior," Pain, 51(1990):75-80.
63 Beecher, "Relationship of significance of wound to pain experienced,"1604-1613.
64 Gøtzsche PC, Nielsen M. "Screening for breast cancer with mammography," Cochrane Database of Systematic Reviews 4 (2009): Art. No.: CD001877. DOI: 10.1002/14651858.CD001877.pub3.
65 Crewdson J., "Rethinking the mammogram guidelines," The Atlantic, November 19, 2009. (Accessed November 23, 2009, at http://www.theatlantic.com/doc/200911u/mammograms.)
66 "Screening for breast cancer: U.S. Preventive Services Task Force recommendation statement," Ann Intern Med 151 (2009):716-26 Medline; http://www.uspreventiveservicestaskforce.org/uspstf/uspsbrca.htm
67 http://well.blogs.nytimes.com/2012/04/18/why-was-warren-buffett-screened-for-prostate-cancer/?hpw
68 "Screening for Prostate Cancer: A Review of the Evidence for the U.S. Preventive Services Task Force," Ann Intern Med., October 7, 2011.
69 http://www.medscape.com/viewarticle/751159_print
70http://www.nytimes.com/2010/03/10/opinion/10Ablin.html?scp=1&sq=Richard%20Ablin&st=cse
71http://www.nytimes.com/2010/03/10/opinion/10Ablin.html?scp=1&sq=Richard%20Ablin&st=cse
72 http://abcnews.go.com/blogs/health/2011/10/07/psa-tests-for-prostate-cancer-more-harm-than-good/; http://online.wsj.com/article/SB10001424052702304707604577422090223876520.html#articleTabs%3Darticle%26commentId%3D4217789%253Fmod%253Ddjemcomnewtrackedcomment
73 "Prostate Cancer Screening—The Evidence, the Recommendations, and the Clinical Implications," JAMA 306,24 (2011):2721-2722; http://www.uspreventiveservicestaskforce.org/uspstf/uspsprca.htm
74 http://en.wikipedia.org/wiki/MMR_vaccine_controversy
75 http://choosingwisely.org/?page_id=13
76 Weinstein, J., et al, "Surgical vs Nonoperative Treatment for Lumbar Disk Herniation," JAMA, 296,20(2006):2441-2450.
77 McQuay, H., "Chapter 31, Drug treatment of chronic pain," *Evidence Based Chronic Pain Management*, (2010).
78 Botwin KP, et al. "Complications of fluoroscopically guided interlaminar cervical

epidural injections,"Arch Phys Med Rehabil 84 (2003):627–633.

79 Vad VB, B., et al., "Transforaminal epidural steroid injections in lumbosacral radiculopathy," Spine 27,1 (2002)11–16; Karppinen J, et al."Periradicular infiltration for sciatica: a randomized controlled trial," Spine 26,9(2001):1059–1067; Karppinen J, et al., "Cost effectiveness of periradicular infiltration for sciatica," Spine 26,23(2001)2587–2595.

80 Riew KD,et al. "The effect of nerve-root injections on the need for operative treatment of lumbar radicular pain: A prospective, randomized, controlled, double-blind study," J Bone Joint Surg (Am) 82,A11(2000):1589–1593; Riew KD, et al. "Nerve root blocks in the treatment of lumbar radicular pain," J Bone Joint Surg (Am) 88,A8(2006):1722–1725.

81 Weinstein, J., et al, "Surgical vs Nonoperative Treatment for Lumbar Disk Herniation," JAMA, 296,20(2006):2441-2450.

82 Manchikanti L. "The growth of interventional pain management in the new millennium: a critical analysis of utilization in the Medicare population," Pain Physician 2004; 7: 465– 482.

83 Jensen, M., "Magnetic resonant imaging of the lumbar spine in people without back pain," N Engl J Med, 331(1994):69-73.

84 Dreyfus P, Dreyer S. "Lumbar zygapophysial joint (facet) injections," Spine J 2003; 3: 50S–9S; Berven S, et al. "The lumbar zygapo- physeal (facet) joints: a role in the pathogenesis of spinal pina syndromes and degenerative spondylolisthesis," Semin Neurol 2002; 22: 187–195; Resnick D, et al. "American Association of Neurological Surgeons/ Congress of Neurological Surgeons. Guidelines for the performance of fusion procedures for degenerative disease of the lumbar spine Part 13: Injection therapies, low- back pain, and lumbar fusion," J Neurosurg Spine 2005; 2: 707–715.

85 Dragovich, A., Cohen, S.,"Interventional therapies," Evidence Based Chronic Pain Management, (2010):384.

86 Luukkainen R, et al.,"Periarticular corticosteroid treatment of the sacroiliac joint in patients with seronegative spondyloarthropathy," Clin Exp Rheumatol 1999; 17: 88–90; Fischer T, et al., "Sacroiliitis in children with spondyloarthropathy: therapeutic effect of CT-guided intra-articular corticosteroid injection (in German)," Rofo 2003; 175: 814–821; Luukkainen R, et al., "Efficacy of periarticular corticosteroid treatment of the sacroiliac joint in non-spondyloarthropathic patients with chronic low back pain in the region of the sacroiliac joint,"Clin Exp Rheumatol 2002; 20: 52–54; Maugars Y, et al., "Assessment of the efficacy of sacroiliac corticosteroid injections in spondyloarthropathies: a double-blind study," Br J Rheumatol, 35(1996):767–770.

87 Wilco, P., et al., "Surgery versus Prolonged Conservative Treatment for Sciatica," N Engl J Med, 356(2007):2245-56.

88 Ioannidis JPA. "Why most published research findings are false," PLoS Med 2005; 2: e124. www.plosmedicine.org.

89 http://www.thecochranelibrary.com/

90 Kraus VB: "Biomarkers and osteoarthritis." In Ginsberg GS, Willard HF (eds): *Genomic and Personalized Medicine.* (Maryland Heights, MO, Academic Press).

91 Kraus VB, Nevitt M, Sandell LJ. "Summary of the OA biomarkers workshop 2009--biochemical biomarkers: biology, validation, and clinical studies,"

Osteoarthritis Cartilage. 2010;18(6):742-745.

92 Deane KD, Norris JM, Holers VM. "Preclinical rheumatoid arthritis: identification, evaluation, and future directions for investigation," Rheum Dis Clin North Am. 2010;36(2):213-241.

93 American College of Rheumatology Subcommittee on Osteoarthritis Guidelines. Recommendations for the medical management of osteoarthritis of the hip and knee: 2000 update. American College of Rheumatology Subcommittee on Osteoarthritis Guidelines. Arthritis Rheum. 2000;43(9):1905-1915; American College of Rheumatology Ad Hoc Group on Use of Selective and Nonselective Nonsteroidal Antiinflammatory Drugs. Recommendations for use of selective and nonselective nonsteroidal antiinflammatory drugs: an American College of Rheumatology white paper. Arthritis Rheum. 2008;59(8):1058-1073; Jordan KM, Arden NK, Doherty M, et al. "EULAR Recommendations 2003: an evidence based approach to the management of knee osteoarthritis: Report of a Task Force of the Standing Committee for International Clinical Studies Including Therapeutic Trials (ESCISIT)," Ann Rheum Dis. 2003;62(12):1145-1155; Zhang W, Nuki G, Moskowitz RW, et al. "OARSI recommendations for the management of hip and knee osteoarthritis: part III: changes in evidence following systematic cumulative update of research published through January 2009," Osteoarthritis Cartilage. 2010;18(4):476-499; Towheed TE, Maxwell L, Judd MG, et al. "Acetaminophen for osteoarthritis," Cochrane Database Syst Rev. 2006;(1):CD004257.

94 Zhang, W., et al., "OARSI recommendations for the management of hip and knee osteoarthritis Part III: changes in evidence following systematic cumulative update of research published through January 2009," Osteoarthritis and Cartilage, 18 (2010): 476–499.

95 Dowson, A., "Prevalence and diagnosis of migraine in a primary care setting," Cephalalgia, 22 (2002):590.

96 Lipton, R., "Migraine Diagnosis and Treatment: Results From the American Migraine Study II," Headache: The Journal of Head and Face Pain, 41, 7 (2001): 638-45.

97 First or worst headache, change in headache pattern, abrupt onset, neurological symptoms lasting >1 hour, new headache in patients with cancer, immunosuppression or pregnancy, loss of consciousness, headache triggered by exertion or sex; Kaniecki, R., "Headache Assessment and Management," JAMA, 289, 11 (2003):1430-33.

98 Olesen, J., "The international classification of headache disorders, 2nd edn (ICDH-II)," J Neurol Neurosurg Psychiatry, 75 (2004): 808-81.

99 Ferrari MD, Goadsby PJ, Roon KI, Lipton RB. "Triptans (serotonin, 5-HT1B/1D agonists) in migraine: detailed results and methods of a meta-analysis of 53 trials," Cephalalgia 2002; 22: 633–658.

100 Ferrari MD, Roon KI, Lipton RB, Goadsby PJ. "Oral triptans (serotonin 5-HT1B/!D agonists) in acute migraine: a meta-analysis of 53 trials," Lancet 2001; 358: 1668–1675.

101 S.D. Silberstein, S., "Evidence-based guideline update: Pharmacologic treatment for episodic migraine prevention in adults," Neurology, 78 (2012):1337-1345.

102 Kaniecki, R., "Headache Assessment and Management," JAMA, 289, 11 (2003):1430-33; Snow, V., "Pharmacologic Management of Acute Attacks of

Migraine and Prevention of Migraine Headache," Ann Intern Med, 137, 10 (2002): 840-9.
103 Cady, R., "Effect of early intervention with sumatriptan on migraine pain: Retrospective analyses of data from three clinical trials," Clin Ther, 22, 9 (2000): 1035-48.
104 Kaniecki, R., "Mixing Sumatriptan: A Prospective Study of Stratified Care Using Multiple Formulations," Headache, 41, 9 (2001): 862-66.
105 Harris RE, Clauw DJ: How do we know that the pain in fibromyalgia is "real," Curr Pain Headache Rep 2006, 10:403-407.
106 Wolfe F, Smythe HA, Yunus MB, Bennett RM, Bombardier C, Goldenberg DL, Tugwell P, Campbell SM, Abeles M, Clark P, Fam AG, Farber SJ, Fiechtner JJ, Franklin CM, Gatter RA, Hamaty D, Lessard J, Lichtbroun AS, Masi AT, Mccain GA, Reynolds WJ, Romano TJ, Russell IJ, Sheon RP: "The American College of Rheumatology 1990 Criteria for the Classification of Fibromyalgia. Report of the Multicenter Criteria Committee," Arthritis Rheum 1990, 33:160-172.
107 Arnold LM, Bradley LA, Clauw DJ, Glass JM, Goldenberg DL. "Evaluating and diagnosing fibromyalgia and comorbid psychiatric disorders," J Clin Psychiatry. 2008;69:e28.
108 Drewes AM. "Pain and sleep disturbances with special reference to fibromyalgia and rheumatoid arthritis," Rheumatology (Oxford). 1999;38:1035-1038.
108 Delgado JA, Murali G, Goldberg R. "Sleep disorders in fibromyalgia. Sleep," 2004;27:A339.
108 Khan SA, Goldberg R, Haber A. "Sleep disorders in fibromyalgia," Sleep. 2005;28:A290.
109 Bannwarth B, Blotman F, Roué-Le Lay K, Caubère JP, André E, Taïeb C: "Fibromyalgia syndrome in the general population of France: A prevalence study," Joint Bone Spine 2009, 76:184-187; McNalley JD, Matheson DA, Bakowshy VS: The epidemiology of self-reported fibromyalgia in Canada; Chronic Dis Can 2006, 27:9-16.
110 Bartels EM et al (2009). "Fibromyalgia, diagnosis and prevalence. Are gender differences explainable?", Ugeskr Laeger. 171 (49): 3588–92.
111 Yunus MB, Aldag JC. "Restless legs syndrome and leg cramps in fibromyalgia syndrome: a controlled study," BMJ. 1996;312:1339; Viola-Saltzman M, Watson NF, Bogart A, Goldberg J, Buchwald D. "High prevalence of restless legs syndrome among patients with fibromyalgia: a controlled cross-sectional study," J Clin Sleep Med. 2010;6:423-427.
112 Burckhardt CS, Goldenberg D, Crofford L, et al. "Guideline for the management of fibromyalgia syndrome. Pain in adults and children," APS Clinical Practice Guideline Series No. 4. Glenview, Ill: American Pain Society; 2005.
Häuser W, Petzke F, Sommer C. "Comparative efficacy and harms of duloxetine, milnacipran, and pregabalin in fibromyalgia syndrome," J Pain. 2010;11:505-521. Epub 2010 Apr 24. Williams DA, Cary MA, Groner KH, et al. "Improving physical functional status in patients with fibromyalgia: a brief cognitive behavioral intervention," J Rheumatol. 2002;29:1280-1286.
113 Häuser W, Petzke F, Sommer C. "Comparative efficacy and harms of duloxetine, milnacipran, and pregabalin in fibromyalgia syndrome," J Pain. 2010;11:505-521.

114 Häuser, W., "Guidelines on the management of fibromyalgia syndrome – A systematic review," European Journal of Pain, 14 (2010): 5–10; Häuser, W., *Evidence-Based Chronic Pain Management* (West Sussex: BMJ Publishing Group, 2010), 121-133.

115 Mailis-Gagnon A, Micholson K. "Nondermatomal somatosensory deficits: overview of unexplainable negative sensory phenomena in chronic pain patients," Curr Opin Anaesthesiol. 2010;23:593-597.

116 Dworkin RH, Backonja M, Rowbotham MC, et al. "Advances in neuropathic pain. Diagnosis, mechanisms, and treatment recommendations," Arch Neurol. 2003;60:1524-1534.

117 Dworkin RH, O'Connor AB, Backonja M, et al. "Pharmacologic management of neuropathic pain: evidence-based recommendations," Pain. 2007;132:237-251; Gatti A, Sabato AF, Occhioni R, et al. Controlled-release oxycodone and pregabalin in the treatment of neuropathic pain: results of a multicenter Italian study. Eur Neurol. 2009;61:129-137; Keskinbora K, Pekel AF, Aydinli I. "Gabapentin and an opioid combination versus opioid alone for the management of neuropathic cancer pain: a randomized open trial," J Pain Symptom Manage. 2007;34:183-189; Gilron I, Bailey JM, Dongsheng T, et al. "Morphine, gabapentin, or their combination for neuropathic pain," N Eng J Med. 2005;352:1324-1334.

118 Dworkin RH, O'Connor AB, Backonja M, et al. "Pharmacologic management of neuropathic pain: evidence-based recommendations," Pain. 2007;132:237-251.

119 Dubinsky RM, Kabbani H, El-Chami Z, et al. "Practice parameter: treatment of postherpetic neuralgia: an evidence-based report of the Quality Standards Committee of the American Academy of Neurology," Neurology. 2004;63:959-965.

120 Lesser H, Sharma U, LaMoreaux L, Poole RM. "Pregabalin relieves symptoms of painful diabetic neuropathy: a randomized controlled trial," Neurology. 2004;63:2104-2110; Richter RW, Portenoy R, Sharma U, Lamoreaux L, Bockbrader H, Knapp LE. "Relief of painful diabetic peripheral neuropathy with pregabalin: a randomized, placebo controlled trial," J Pain. 2005;6:253-260. Rosenstock J, Tuchman M, LaMoreaux L, Sharma U. "Pregabalin for the treatment of painful diabetic peripheral neuropathy: a double-blind, placebo-controlled trial," Pain. 2004;110:628-638.

121 Bril V, England J, Franklin GM, et al. "Evidence-based guideline: treatment of painful diabetic neuropathy: report of the American Academy of Neurology, the American Association of Neuromuscular and Electrodiagnostic Medicine, and the American Academy of Physical Medicine and Rehabilitation," Neurology. 2011;76:1758-1765; Raskin J, Pritchett YL, Wang F, et al. "A double-blind, randomized multicenter trial comparing duloxetine with placebo in the management of diabetic peripheral neuropathic pain," Pain Med. 2005;6:346-356; Jones VM, Moore KA, Peterson DM. "Capsaicin 8% topical patch (qutenza)-a review of the evidence," J Pain Palliat Care Pharmacother. 2011;25:32-41.

122 Haythornthwaite JA, Benrud-Larson LM. "Psychological assessment and treatment of patients with neuropathic pain," Curr Pain Headache Rep. 2001;5:124-129; Ahn AC, Bennani T, Freeman R, Hamdy O, Kaptchuk TJ. "Two styles of acupuncture for treating painful diabetic neuropathy--a pilot randomized control trial," Acupunct Med. 2007;25:11-17; Abuaisha BB, Costanzi JB, Boulton AJ. "Acupuncture for the treatment of chronic painful peripheral diabetic neuropathy: a

long-term study," Diabetes Res Clin Pract. 1998;39:115-121.

123 Haythornthwaite JA, Benrud-Larson LM. "Psychological assessment and treatment of patients with neuropathic pain," Curr Pain Headache Rep. 2001;5:124-129; Argoff CE. "Review of current guidelines on the care of postherpetic neuralgia," Postgrad Med. 2011;123:134-142.

124 Bril V, England J, Franklin GM, et al. "Evidence-based guideline: treatment of painful diabetic neuropathy: report of the American Academy of Neurology, the American Association of Neuromuscular and Electrodiagnostic Medicine, and the American Academy of Physical Medicine and Rehabilitation," Neurology. 2011;76:1758-1765.

125 McQuay, H., "Chapter 7, Chronic Low Back Pain," *Evidence Based Chronic Pain Management*, (2010).

126 Age of onset <20 or >55 years, Violent trauma, Constant progressive, nonmechanical pain (no relief with bedrest), Thoracic pain, History of malignant tumor, use of corticosteroids, Drug abuse, immunosuppression, HIV, Signs of systemic disease, Unexplained weight loss, Widespread symptomology, Structural deformity, Fever.

127 Heymans, M., et al., "Back Schools for Nonspecific Low Back Pain: A Systematic Review Within the Framework of the Cochrane Collaboration Back Review Group," Spine, 30, 19 (2005): 2153-2163.

128 Nelemans PJ, de Bie RA, de Vet HCW, et al. "Injection therapy for subacute and chronic benign low back pain," The Cochrane Library, Issue 3, 2002. Update Software, Oxford.

129 Hickey RF. "Chronic low back pain: a comparison of diflunisal with paracetamol," NZ Med J 1982; 95(707): 312–314.

130 Nelemans PJ, de Bie RA, de Vet HCW, et al. "Injection therapy for subacute and chronic benign low back pain," The Cochrane Library, Issue 3, 2002. Update Software, Oxford.

131 Hayden JA, van Tulder MW, Tomlinson G. "Systematic review: strategies for using exercise therapy to improve outcomes in chronic low back pain," Ann Intern Med 2005; 142(9): 776–785.

132 Hayden JA, van Tulder MW, Malmivaara AV, Koes BW. "Meta-analysis: exercise therapy for nonspecific low back pain," Ann Intern Med 2005; 142(9): 765–775.

133 Gibson JNA, Ahmed M. "The effectiveness of flexible and rigid supports in patients with lumbar backache," J Orthop Med 2002; 24: 86–9.

134 Ostelo RW, et al., "Behavioural treatment for chronic low- back pain," Cochrane Database Syst Rev, 1(2005). Jan 25;(1): CD002014.

135 Furlan AD, Brosseau L, Imamura M, Irvin E. "Massage for low-back pain: a systematic review within the framework of the Cochrane Collaboration Back Review Group," Spine 2002; 27: 1896–1910.

136 van Tulder MW, Touray T, Furlan AD, Solway S, Bouter LM, Cochrane Back Review Group. "Muscle relaxants for nonspecific low back pain: a systematic review within the framework of the Cochrane Collaboration," Spine 2003; 28(17): 1978–1992.

137 Assendelft WJJ,et al., "Spinal manipulative therapy for low back pain. A meta-analysis of effectiveness relative to other therapies," Ann Intern Med 59, 138 (2003):

871–881.

138 Furlan AD, et al., "Acupuncture and dry-needling for low back pain: an updated systematic review within the framework of the Cochrane Collaboration," Spine ; 30, 8 (2005): 944–963.

139 van Tulder MW, et al., "Conservative treatment of acute and chronic non-specific low back pain: a systematic review of randomized controlled trials of the most common interventions," Spine, 22 (1997): 2128–2156.

140 Browning R, Jackson JF, O'Malley PG. "Cyclobenzaprine and back pain," Arch Intern Med 2001; 161: 1613–1620; Salerno SM, Browning R, Jackson JL. "The effect of antidepressant treatment in chronic back pain: a meta-analysis," Arch Intern Med 2002; 162: 19–24.

141 Clarke JA, van Tulder MW, Blomberg SE, et al. "Traction for low-back pain with or without sciatica," Cochrane Database Syst Rev. 2007 Apr 18; (2): CD003010.

142 Guzman J, Esmail R, Karjalainen K, Malmivaara A, Irvin E, Bombardier C. "Multidisciplinary rehabilitation for chronic low back pain: systematic review," BMJ 2001; 322(7301): 1511–1516.

143 Milne S, Welch V, Brosseau L, Saginur M, Shea B, Tugwell P, Wells G. "Transcutaneous electrical nerve stimulation (TENS) for chronic low back pain," Cochrane Database Syst Rev. 2001; (2): CD003008.

144 Chou,R., "Diagnosis and Treatment of Low Back Pain: A Joint Clinical Practice Guideline," The American College of Physicians and the American Pain Society, 147,7(2007):478-491.

145 Carroll, Lewis. *Alice's Adventures in Wonderland,* (New York:MacMillan. 1865).

146 Kahneman, Daniel. *Thinking, fast and slow.* (New York: Farrar, Straus and Giroux 2011).

147 Alan Watts, Myth of Myself 1958.

148 The Magical Number Seven, Plus or Minus Two: Some Limits on Our Capacity for Processing Information.

149 Williams, D.A., Keefe, F.J.,"Pain beliefs and the use of cognitive-behavioural coping strategies," Pain, 46(1991): 185-190.

150 Arnstein, P., Caudill, M., et al, "Self efficacy as a mediator of the relationship between pain intensity, disability and depression in chronic pain patients," Pain, 80(1999):483- 491.

151 Turk DC, Okifuji A., "Psychological Factors in Chronic Pain: Evolution and Revolution," J of Consulting and clinical Psychology, (2002):678-690.

152 Ballantyne, J.,"Opioid Therapy for Chronic Pain," N Engl J Med, 349,20(2003):1943-1953.

153 Ibid.

154 Savage, S., "Long-term opioid therapy: Assessment of consequences and risks," Journal of Pain and Symptom Management 11(1996):274-286.

155 Ibid.

156 Compton P, Athanasos P, Elashoff D., "Withdrawal hyperalgesia after acute opioid physical dependence in nonaddicted humans: a preliminary study," J Pain 4(2003):511–519.

157 McQuay H. Opioids in pain management. Lancet. 1999;353: 2229–2232.

Mercadante S, Bruera E. "Opioid switching: a systematic and critical review," Cancer Treat Rev. 2006;32:304–315; Brodner RA, Taub A. "Chronic pain exacerbated by long- term narcotic use in patients with non-malignant disease: clinical syndrome and treatment," Mt Sinai J Med. 1978;45: 233–237.

158 Mao J. "Opioid-induced abnormal pain sensitivity: implications in clinical opioid therapy," Pain 2002;100:213-7.

159 Opioid Analgesia: Perspectives on Right Use and Utility, Pain Physician 2007; 10:479-491.

160 Wilder-Smith O, Arendt-Nielsen L. 'Postoperative hyperalgesia: its clinical importance and relevance" Anesthesiology. 2006; 104:601–607. Mitra S, Sinatra R. "Perioperative management of acute pain in the opioid-dependent patient," Anesthesiology. 2004;101:212–227; Rapp S, Ready L, Nessly M. "Acute pain management in patients with prior opioid consumption: a case-controlled retrospective review," Pain. 1995;61:195–201; "Efficacy of Opioids for Chronic Pain: A Review of the Evidence," Jane C. Ballantyne, Clin J Pain ! Volume 24, Number 6, July/August 2008; Mercadante S, Bruera E. Opioid switching: a systematic and critical review. Cancer Treat Rev. 2006;32:304–315; Brodner RA, Taub A. "Chronic pain exacerbated by longterm narcotic use in patients with non-malignant disease: clinical syndrome and treatment," Mt Sinai J Med. 1978;45: 233–237; McQuay H. "Opioids in pain management," Lancet. 1999;353: 2229–2232.

161 Pasternak GW. "The pharmacology of mu analgesics: from patients to genes," Neuroscientist 2001;7:220-31.

162 Brodner RA, Taub A. "Chronic pain exacerbated by long- term narcotic use in patients with non-malignant disease: clinical syndrome and treatment," Mt Sinai J Med. 1978;45: 233–237; Devulder J. "Hyperalgesia induced by high-dose intrathecal sufentanil in neuropathic pain," J Neurosurg Anesthesiol. 1997;9: 146–148; Chu LF, Clark D, Angst M. "Opioid tolerance and ,"hyperalgesia in chronic pain patients after one month of oral morphine therapy: a preliminary prospective study. J Pain. 2006;7:43–48; "Savage SR. Long-term opioid therapy: assessment of consequences and risks," J Pain Symptom Manage. 1996;11:274–286.

163 Katz N., "Methodological issues in clinical trials of opioids for chronic pain," Neurology, 65(2005):S32–S49; Ballantyne, J.,"Efficacy of Opioids for Chronic Pain: A Review of the Evidence," Clin J Pain (2008;24:469–478).

164 Ballantyne, J.,"Efficacy of Opioids for Chronic Pain: A Review of the Evidence," Clin J Pain (2008;24:469–478).

165 Kalso E, Edwards J, Moore R, et al., "Opioids in chronic non-cancer pain: systematic review of efficacy and safety," Pain, 112(2004):372–380; Moore RA, McQuay HJ., "Prevalence of opioid adverse events in chronic non-malignant pain: systematic review of randomised trials of oral opioids," Arthritis Res Ther., 7(2005):R1046–R1051; Furlan AD, Sandoval JA, Mailis-Gagnon A, et al., "Opioids for chronic non-cancer pain: a meta-analysis of effectiveness and side effects," Can Med Assoc J., 174(2006):1589–1594.

166 Mendelson, M., "Effects of heroin and methadone on plasma cortisol and testosterone," J Pharmacol Exp Ther 1975 195:296-302; Ballantyne, J., "Opioid Therapy for Chronic Pain," N Engl J Med (2003) 349:1943-53; "Critical issues on opioids in chronic non-cancer pain: an epidemiological study."; J Eriksen, Pain, 2006; Daniell, HW., "Hypogonadism in men consuming sustained-action oral

opioids." J Pain 2002 3:377-384.

167 Ballantyne, J., "Efficacy of Opioids for Chronic Pain: A Review of the Evidence," Clin J Pain, 24(2008):469–478.

168 Ballantyne JC., "Opioids for chronic pain: taking stock," Pain, 125(2006):3–4; Chou R., Clark, E., Helfand, M., "Comparative efficacy and safety of long-acting oral opioids for chronic non-cancer pain: a systematic review," J Pain Symptom Manage, 26(2003):1026–1048.

169 Eriksen J, Sjogren P, Bruera E, et al. "Critical issues on opioids in chronic non-cancer pain. An epidemiological study," Pain 125(2006):172–179.

170 Eriksen J, Sjogren P, Bruera E, et al. "Critical issues on opioids in chronic non-cancer pain. An epidemiological study," Pain. 2006; 125:172–179; Joranson DE. "Improving availability of opioid pain medications: testing the principle of balance in Latin America," J Palliat Med. 2004;7:105–114.

171 "Critical issues on opioids in chronic non-cancer pain: an epidemiological study."; J Eriksen, Pain, 2006.

172 Addiction: Why Can't They Just Stop (c) 2007 Rodale, Inc.; Cami J, Farre M. "Drug addiction," N Engl J Med. 2003;349: 975–986; Koob G, Le Moal M. "Drug addiction, dysregulation of reward, and allostasis," Neuropharmcology. 2001;24:97–129; Koob G, Le Moal M. "Drug abuse: hedonic homeostatic dysregulation," Science. 1997;278:52–58.

173 http://www.nytimes.com/2011/07/11/health/11addictions.html?hp

174 Ballantyne, J., "Opioid Analgesia: Perspectives on right use and utility," Pain Physician, 10(2007):479-491.

175 Schofferman, J., "Long term use of opioid analgesics for the treatment of chronic pain of nonmalignant origin," J Pain and Symp Man, 8,5(1993):286.

176 Schofferman, J., "Long term use of opioid analgesics for the treatment of chronic pain of nonmalignant origin," J Pain and Symp Man, 8,5(1993):279-288.

177 http://www.nytimes.com/2002/01/22/health/personal-health-misunderstood-opioids-and-needless-pain.html?scp=4&sq=opioids&st=cse

[178] https://www.nytimes.com/2017/09/04/well/opioids-arent-the-only-pain-drugs-to-fear.html

179 Levine, J. D., Gordon, N. C., Smith, R.,&Fields, H. L., "Analgesic responses to morphine and placebo in individuals with postoperative pain," Pain, 10(1981):379-389.

180 Levine, J. D.,&Gordon, N. C., "Influence of the method of drug administration on analgesic response," Nature, 312(1984):755-756.

181 Buchalew, L.W. And K.E. Coffield, "An investigation of drug expectancy as a function of colour, size and preparation," J. Clin Pharmacol, 2(1982):245-248.

182 Thomas, K. B., "General practice consultations: Is there any point in being positive?," British Medical Journal, 294(1987):1200-1202.

183 Fabrizzio Benedetti, "How the Doctor's Words Affect the Patient's Brain," Evaluation and the Health Profession, 25(2002): 371.

184 Ibid.; p.372

185 http://www.washingtonpost.com/ac2/wp-dyn/A2709-2002Apr29

186 Ibid.

187 Flaten MA, Simonsen T, Olsen H., "Drug-related information generates placebo and nocebo responses that modify the drug response," Psychosom Med,

61(1999):250–255.

188 Barsky AJ, Saintfort R, Rogers MP, Borus JF., "Nonspecific medication side effects and the nocebo phenomenon," JAMA, 287(2002):622–627.

189 http://www.washingtonpost.com/ac2/wp-dyn/A2709-2002Apr29

190 Amanzio, M., Pollo, A., Maggi, G.,&Benedetti, F., "Response variability to analgesics:A role for nonspecific activation of endogenous opioids," Pain, 90(2001):205-215.

191 Benedetti, F., "Cholecystokinin type-A and type-B receptors and their modulation of opioid analgesia," News in Physiological Sciences, 12(1997):263-268.

192 Fabrizio Benedetti, "How the Doctor's Words Affect the Patient's Brain," Eval Health Prof, 25(2002): 382.

193 Shetty, N., et al., "The placebo response in Parkinson's disease. Parkinson study group," Clinical Neuropharmacology, 22(1999): 207-212.

194 Goetz, C. G., et al., "Objective changes in motor function during placebo treatment in Parkinson's disease," Neurology, 54(2000): 710-714.

195 60 Minutes, "Treating Depression," Feb. 19, 2012; http://www.cbsnews.com/8301-18560_162-57380893/treating-depression-is-there-a-placebo-effect/

196 Kirkley A, Birmingham TB, Litchfield RB, et al. (September 2008). "A randomized trial of arthroscopic surgery for osteoarthritis of the knee," N. Engl. J. Med. 359 (11): 1097–107.

197 http://www.nytimes.com/2008/09/11/health/research/11knee.html

198 60 Minutes, "Treating Depression," Feb. 19, 2012; http://www.cbsnews.com/8301-18560_162-57380893/treating-depression-is-there-a-placebo-effect/

199 Fabrizio Benedetti, "How the Doctor's Words Affect the Patient's Brain," Eval Health Prof, 25(2002): 382.

200 Luana Colloca and Fabrizio Benedetti, "Nocebo hyperalgesia: how anxiety is turned into pain," Curr Opin Anaesthesiol, 20(2007):437.

201 National Institute on Drug Abuse. National household survey on drug abuse: highlights 1991. Washington DC: US GovernmentPrinting Office; 1991.

202 http://drugwarfacts.org/cms/files/Drug-Rankings-by-Harm.pdf

203 Rowbotham MC, et al. "Treatment response in antidepressant -naïve postherpetic neuralgia patients: double-blind, randomized trial," J Pain 6 (2005):741-746.

204 Dworkin RH, et al. "Advances in neuropathic pain: diagnosis, mechanisms, and treatment recommendations," Arch Neurol 60 (2003):1524-1534.

205 Dworkin RH, et al. "Recommendations for the pharmacological management of neuropathic pain: an overview and literature update," Mayo Clin Proc 85 (2010): S3-S14.

206 Rowbotham MC, et al, "Lidocaine patch: double-blind controlled study of a new treatment method for post-herpetic neuralgia," Pain 65 (1996): 39-44.

207 Wallace M, et al, "A capsaicin 8% patch for the management of postherpetic neuralgia," Expert Rev Neurother 11 (2011):15-27.

208 Boureau F, et al, "Tramadol in post-herpetic neuralgia: a randomized, double-blind, placebo-controlled trial," Pain 104 (2003): 323-331.

209 Hanson, *Coping with Chronic Pain*, v.

210 World Health Organisation International Classification of Functioning, Disability and Health 2000.
211 Fritz, J.M., George, S.Z., "The role of fear avoidance beliefs in acute low back pain: relationships with current and future disability and work status," Pain, 94(2001):7-15.
212 Bortz, W.M., "The disuse syndrome," Western Journal of Medicine, (1984):691-698.
213 Main, C., Watson, P., "Guarded movements: development of chronicity," Pain, 4(1996):163-170.
214 Vlaeyen JWS Linton SJ., "Fear avoidance and its consequences in chronic musculoskeletal pain: a state of the art," Pain, 85(2000):317-332.
215 http://www.childbirthconnection.org/article.asp?ck=10456
216 Moseley JB, O'Malley K, Petersen NJ, et al. (July 2002). "A controlled trial of arthroscopic surgery for osteoarthritis of the knee," N. Engl. J. Med. 347 (2): 81–8.
217 Kirkley A, Birmingham TB, Litchfield RB, et al. (September 2008). "A randomized trial of arthroscopic surgery for osteoarthritis of the knee," N. Engl. J. Med. 359 (11): 1097–107.
218 http://www.nytimes.com/2008/09/11/health/research/11knee.html
219 https://www.nytimes.com/2016/08/04/upshot/the-right-to-know-that-an-operation-is-next-to-useless.html
220 Waddell, G., "A New Clinical Model for the Treatment of Low-Back Pain," Spine 12 ( ):632.
221 Hofstee DJ, Gijtenbeek JM, Hoogland PH, et al. "Westeinde sciatica trial: randomized controlled study of bed rest and physiotherapy for acute sciatica," J Neurosurg 2002;96:Suppl 1:45-9.
222 Awad JN, Moskovich R. 'Lumbar disc herniations: surgical versus nonsurgical treatment,' Clin Orthop Relat Res 2006; 443:183-97.
223 Weber H. Lumbar disc herniation: a controlled, prospective study with ten years of observation. Spine 1983;8:131-40.
224http://online.wsj.com/article/SB1000142405311190410670457658262167735450 8.html?KEYWORDS=spinal+fusion+was+the+16th+most+common
225http://online.wsj.com/article/SB1000142405311190410670457658262167735450 8.html?KEYWORDS=spinal+fusion+was+the+16th+most+common
226 Wilco, P., et al., "Surgery versus Prolonged Conservative Treatment for Sciatica," N Engl J Med, 356(2007):2245-56.
227 Osterman H, et al., "Effectiveness of microdiscectomy for lumbar disc herniation: a randomized controlled trial with 2 years of follow-up," Spine 31(2006):2409-2414.
228 Deyo, R., et al., "Trends, Major Medical Complications, and Charges Associated With Surgery for Lumbar Spinal Stenosis in Older Adults," JAMA, 303,13(2010).
229 Jensen, M., "Magnetic resonant imaging of the lumbar spine in people without back pain," N Engl J Med, 331(1994):69-73.
230 Waddell, *Model for the Treatment of Low-Back Pain*, 637.
231 North, R., "Spinal cord stimulation versus repeated lumbosacral spine surgery for chronic pain: A Randomized, Controlled Trial," Neurosurgery, 56 (2005): 98-107.
232 North RB, Ewend MG, Lawton MT, Kidd DH, Piantadosi S. 'Failed back

surgery syndrome: 5-year follow-up after spinal cord stimulator implantation," Neurosurgery. 1991;28:692-699; Ohnmeiss DD, Rashbaum RF, Bogdanffy GM. "Prospective outcome evaluation of spinal cord stimulation in patients with intractable leg pain," Spine. 1996;21:1344-1350; De La Porte C, Van de Kelft E. "Spinal cord stimulation in failed back surgery syndrome," Pain. 1993;52:55-61; Turner JA, Loeser JD, Bell KG. "Spinal cord stimulation for chronic low back pain: a systematic literature synthesis," Neurosurgery. 1995;37:1088-1095.

233 Grabow TS, T PK, Srinivasa N. Raja M. "Spinal cord stimulation for complex regional pain syndrome: an evidence- based medicine review of the literature," Clin J Pain 2003; 19: 371–383; Mailis-Gagnon A, Furlan MD, Sandoval JA, Taylor RS. "Spinal cord stimulation for chronic pain," Cochrane Database of Systematic Reviews 2004, Issue 3; Cameron T. "Safety and efficacy of spinal cord stimula- tion for the treatment of chronic pain: a 20-year literature review," J Neurosurg 2004; 100(3 suppl): 254–267. Kemler MA, Reulen JP, van Kleef M, Barendse GA, van den Wildenberg FA, Spaans F. "Thermal thresholds in complex regional pain syndrome type I: sensitivity and repeatability of the methods of limits and levels," Clin Neurophysiol. 2000;111:1561-1568.

234 North RB, Wetzel FT. "Spinal cord stimulation for chronic pain of spinal origin: a valuable long-term solution," Spine. 2002;27:2584-2591.

235 Popenay CA, Alo KM. "Peripheral neurostimulation for the treatment of chronic disabling transformed migraine," Headache. 2003;43:369-375.

236 Mannheimer C, Eliasson T, Augustinsson LE, et al. "Electrical stimulation versus coronary artery bypass surgery in severe angina pectoris: the ESPY study," Circulation. 1998;97:1157-1163.

237 Ballantyne JC, Carwood C. "Comparative efficacy of epi-dural, subarachnoid, and intracerebroventricular opioids in patients with pain due to cancer," Cochrane Database of Systematic Reviews 2005, Issue 2. Art. No.: CD005178.

238 Anderson VC, Burchiel KJ. "A prospective study of long- term intrathecal morphine in the management of chronic nonmalignant pain," Neurosurgery 1999; 44: 289–300; Hassenbusch SJ, Portenoy RK, Cousins M. "Polyanalgesic consensus conference 2003: an update on the management of pain by intraspinal drug delivery – report of an expert panel," J Pain Symptom Manage 2004; 276: 540–563; Angel IF, Gould HJ, Carey ME. "Intrathecal morphine pump as a treatment option in chronic pain of nonmalig- nant origin," Surg Neurol 1998; 49: 92–98; Kumar K, Kelly M, Pirlot T. "Continuous intrathecal morphine treatment for chronic pain of nonmalignant etiology: long-term benefits and efficacy," Surg Neurol 2001; 55: 79–86.

239 Holroyd KA, Penzien DB. "Pharmacological versus non-pharmacological prophylaxis of recurrent migraine headache: a meta-analytic review of clinical trials," Pain, 42 (1990): 1–13.

240 Kwon YD, Pittler MH, Ernst E. "Acupuncture for peripheral joint osteoarthritis: a systematic review and meta-analysis," Rheumatology (Oxford) 2006; 45(11): 1331–1337.

241 Long L. "Herbal medicines for the treatment of osteoarthri- tis a systematic review," Rheumatology 2001; 40: 779–793.

242 Soeken KL, Lee WL, Bausell RB, Agelli M, Berman BM. "Safety and efficacy of S-adenosylmethionine (SAMe) for osteoarthritis," J Fam Pract 2002; 51(5): 425–

430.

243 Müller H, de Toledo FW, Resch KL. "Fasting followed by vegetarian diet in patients with rheumatoid arthritis: a systematic review," Scand J Rheumatol 2001; 30: 1–10.

244 Fortin PR, Lew RA, Liang MH, Wright EA, Beckett LA, Chalmers TC, et al. "Validation of a meta-analysis: the effects of fish oil in rheumatoid arthritis," J Clin Epidemiol 1995; 48: 1379–1390.

245 Han A, Judd M, Welch V, Wu T, Tugwell P, Wells GA. "Tai chi for treating rheumatoid arthritis," Cochrane Database of Systematic Reviews 2004, Issue 3. Art. No.: CD004849. DOI:10.1002/14651858.CD004849.

246 Mongomery GH, David D, Winkel G, Silverstein JH, Bovbjerg DH. "The effectiveness of adjunctive hypnosis with surgical patients: a meta-analysis," Anesth Analg 2002; 94:1639–1645.

247 Bjordal JM, Johnson MI, Ljunggreen AE. "Transcutaneous electrical nerve stimulation (TENS) can reduce postoperative analgesic consumption. A meta-analysis with assess- ment of optimal treatment parameters for postoperative pain," Eur J Pain 2003; 7(2): 181–188.

248 Ernst E. "Complementary and alternative medicine," In: *Dukes MNG (ed) Meyler's Side Effects of Drugs*, vols 2 and 3. Elsevier, Edinburgh, 2006.

249 McQuay, H., "Chapter 31, Drug treatment of chronic pain," *Evidence Based Chronic Pain Management*, (2010).

250 https://www.nytimes.com/2017/08/01/well/live/the-secret-life-of-pain.html?mcubz=0

251 Hanson, "Coping with Chronic Pain," 36.

252 Joshua Foer, *Moonwalking with Einstein* (New York, NY:Penguin Group 2011).

253 Morris, D., *Intractable pain and the perception of time: every patient is an anecdote* (Charlottesville, University of Virginia).

254 https://www.nytimes.com/2017/04/25/well/family/womens-friendships-in-sickness-and-in-health.html?mcubz=0

255 Paul Martin, *The Healing Mind* (Thomas Dunes Books, 1997).

256 Paul Martin, *The Sickening Mind* (Harper Collins, 1997): 157.

257 Social security online: The Red Book 2011.

258 http://www.hawking.org.uk/index.php/disability

259 Moore, *Dark Nights of the Soul* (New York, NY: Penguin Group 2005).

260 http://www.nyaap.org/jung-lexicon/n

261 John Daido Loori, *Mountain Records of Zen Talks* (Boston: Shambhala, 1988), p. 21

262 C. Jung, "The Psychology of the Transference," CW 16, par. 455.

263 Oscar Wilde, *De Profundis*.

264 http://spiritlibrary.com/eckhart-tolle/eckhart-on-the-dark-night-of-the-soul

265 Claire Scobie (2003-08-31). Why now is bliss. Telegraph Magazine. Retrieved on 2010-2-2.

266 Victor Frankl, *Man's Search for Meaning* (New York, NY: Simon and Schuster, 1984)

267 Ibid., p.82.

268 Ibid., p.84.

269 Ibid., p.87-88.

270 Ibid., p.86.

271 Ibid., p.104.

272 Ibid., p.12.

273 Ibid., p.41.

274 McCracken, L., "Learning to live with the pain: acceptance of pain predicts adjustment in persons with chronic pain," Pain 74 (1998): 21.

McCracken, L., et al., "A prospective study of acceptance of pain and patient functioning with chronic pain," Pain 118 (2005): 164.

275 McCracken, L., "Learning to live with the pain," 21-22.

276 Ibid., p.21-27; McCracken, , "A prospective study of acceptance of pain and patient functioning with chronic pain," Pain 118 (2005): 164-169.

[277] Aaron Swartz (R.I.P.), weblog.

[278] Risdon, A., "How can we learn to live with pain? A Q-methodological analysis of the diverse understandings of acceptance of chronic pain," Social Science & Medicine 56 (2003): 375–386.

About the Author:

I write under a pseudonym because I value my privacy. I'm a physician; I have chronic pains; I have something to share with the chronic pain community. The rest is but pabulum.

HMoody.Truce@gmail.com

www.ingramcontent.com/pod-product-compliance
Lightning Source LLC
Chambersburg PA
CBHW071301220526

45468CB00001B/229

9 781981 611324